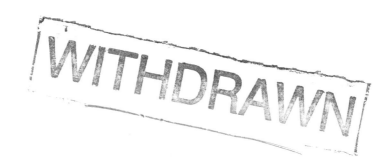

PHARMACOLOGY - RESEARCH, SAFETY TESTING AND REGULATION

PHARMACEUTICAL FORMULATION AND MEDICINAL CHEMISTRY

MECHANISMS, DEVELOPMENTS AND TREATMENTS

PHARMACOLOGY - RESEARCH, SAFETY TESTING AND REGULATION

Additional books in this series can be found on Nova's website
under the Series tab.

Additional e-books in this series can be found on Nova's website
under the e-book tab.

PHARMACOLOGY - RESEARCH, SAFETY TESTING AND REGULATION

PHARMACEUTICAL FORMULATION AND MEDICINAL CHEMISTRY

MECHANISMS, DEVELOPMENTS AND TREATMENTS

BRUCE MOORE
EDITOR

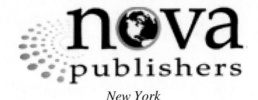

New York

Library of Congress Cataloging-in-Publication Data

ISBN: 978-1-63484-082-8

Library of Congress Control Number: 2015955196

Published by Nova Science Publishers, Inc. † *New York*

CONTENTS

PREFACE

This book reviews research on pharmaceutical formulation and medicinal chemistry. It begins with a summary of old and new discoveries on therapeutic applications of the A3 adenosine receptor in inflammation and cancer, and highlights the most important agonists and antagonists developed for the A3 adenosine receptor, explicitly those in clinical trials for the treatment of inflammation and/or cancer. The next chapter addresses and highlights the different inhibitions against metastases *in vivo* and molecular mechanisms of action *in vitro* of Biz compounds especially relating to the inhibitory efficacies against tumor metastasis and other important clinical utilizations including inhibitory pathways against angiogenesis, topoisomerase II, calmodulin, sialic acid, fibrinogen, drug combinations, medicinal chemistry, cell-movement and so on. Chapter three focuses on concepts of isosterism and bioisosterism in modern medicinal chemistry. The final chapter discusses the determination of L-Dopa in pharmaceutical formulations with a glassy carbon electrode (GCE) modified with cobalt phthalocyanine (CoPc) adsorbed on multi-walled carbon nanotubes (MWCN).

Chapter 1 – A_3 adenosine receptor is a G protein-coupled receptor belonging to P1 family of purinergic receptors. It is widely distributed in human organs and tissues with various expression levels. In particular, A_3 adenosine receptor is highly expressed in several immune cells and cancer cell lines. For this reason, its modulation is intensively studied for the involvement in inflammation and cancer. Ligands (agonists and antagonists) presenting high affinity and selectivity for the A_3 adenosine receptor are essential for determining the role of such receptor in these pathophysiological conditions and, eventually, for the development of potential drugs for their treatment. In this review the authors summarize old and new discoveries on therapeutic applications of the A_3 adenosine receptor in inflammation and cancer, and highlight the most important agonists and antagonists developed for the A_3 adenosine receptor, explicitly those in clinical trials for the treatment of inflammation and/or cancer.

Chapter 2 – This chapter focuses on concepts of isosterism and bioisosterism in modern medicinal chemistry. Drug design and development aspects are illustrated by applying these concepts to the construction of potent enzyme inhibitors. Particular attention is devoted to bioisosteric modifications of the purine scaffold contributing to the molecular diversity and improvements of pharmacodynamic and pharmacokinetic parameters of compounds. The scope of this chapter covers heterocyclic systems generated by various aza- / deaza-replacements of the purine ring atoms. The success of the bioisosterism strategy in the development of clinically useful enzyme inhibitors, constructed on the purine related heterocyclic systems, is exemplified by several important drugs. Sildenafil, inhibiting cGMP-specific phosphodiesterase type 5, has been a blockbuster drug since its launch to the market. It was followed by further isosteric modifications of the ring system that resulted in the development of another representative of this class, vardenafil. Allopurinol, inhibiting one of the key purine catabolizing enzymes – xanthine oxidase, has been a gold standard of chronic gout therapy for more than 50 years. Examples of other drugs, drug candidates, and lead compounds are also discussed in the context of recent trends in the enzyme inhibitor research.

Chapter 3 – A new sensitive voltammetric sensor was developed for electrochemical determination of L-Dopa in pharmaceutical formulations with a glassy carbon electrode (GCE) modified with cobalt phthalocyanine (CoPc) adsorbed on multi-walled carbon nanotubes (MWCN). The electrochemical characterization was performed by Scanning Electron Microscopy (SEM) and Fourier Transform Infrared Spectroscopy (FT-IR). The results have shown that MWCN and CoPc form a composite material without formation of large agglomerates. An estimation of the kinetic parameters α (charge transfer coefficient) and κ (heterogeneous transfer rate constant) was carried out using the Laviron's model resulting in $\alpha = 0.54$ and $\kappa = 22.55$ s^{-1}. These results suggest that the GCE immobilized with CoPc forms a quasi-reversible with high transfer speed response. Thus demonstrating that the sensor is kinetically viable for electrooxidation of CoPc, enabling its use as a catalyst for redox processes of various electroactive species. The optimized conditions of the developed system were: MWCN (2.0 mg.mL^{-1}) and CoPc (2.0 mg.mL^{-1}) in 0.1 mol.L^{-1} pH 7.5 phosphate buffered saline. The operational parameters of electroanalytical DPV and SWV were optimized, and the DPV showed higher sensitivity. Therefore the DPV was chosen for the determination of L-Dopa in the pharmaceutical formulation. An analytical curve was made showing a linear response over the concentration range from 10 to 80 μmol.L^{-1}, with R = 0.999. The *limit* of *detection* (LOD) and the *limit* of *quantification* (*LOQ*) obtained was equal to 3.7636 and 12.545 μmol.L^{-1}, respectively. The validation of the proposed electroanalytical method for the determination of L-Dopa was performed according to ANVISA. The precision and accuracy values obtained by *validate* the *method*, were less than 5% maximum recommended by Resolution No. 899 of ANVISA. Therefore, proposed method for determination of L-Dopa was considered accurate and able to be applied to real samples. The developed sensor applied in real samples presented a good recovery with values between 98.50, 98.64% 99.18%, attesting the accuracy of the procedure.

Chapter 4 – Bisdioxopiperazine compounds, including ICRF-154 and razoxane (ICRF-159, Raz), are anticancer agents developed in the UK in 1969. Novel discoveries and debates about these compounds have been frequently reported worldwide, especially the antimetastatic activity and detoxicatative for anticancer anthrocyclines. Furthermore three bisdioxopiperazine derivatives (Biz compounds), bimolane (Bim), probimane (Pro) and MST-16, have been synthesized at the Shanghai Institute of Materia Medica, Chinese Academy of Sciences, PR China after 1980. Since cancer metastasis, the deadliest pathologic feature of cancers has been the main obstacle in cancer therapy, antimetastatic therapeutic efficacies and mechanisms of action about Biz compounds are of significant clinical interests of all time. This review addresses and highlights the different inhibitions against metastases *in vivo* and molecular mechanisms of action *in vitro* of Biz compounds especially relating to the inhibitory efficacies against tumor metastasis and other important clinical utilizations including inhibitory pathways against angiogenesis, topoisomerase II, calmodulin, sialic acid, fibrinogen, drug combinations, medicinal chemistry, cell-movement and so on.

Since 90% cancer deaths are caused by neoplasm metastasis and cancer stem cells, the systematic exploration of antimetastatic activity and mechanisms of action for Biz compounds seems to be a shortcut for a final solution of cancer therapy in the future.

In: Pharmaceutical Formulation
Editor: Bruce Moore

ISBN: 978-1-63484-082-8
© 2015 Nova Science Publishers, Inc.

Chapter 1

A_3 ADENOSINE RECEPTOR LIGANDS IN THE TREATMENT OF INFLAMMATION AND CANCER

Cheong Siew Lee[1], Federico Stephanie[2*], Tan Boon Wu Aaron [3], Spalluto Giampiero[2] and Pastorin Giorgia[3]*

[1]Department of Pharmaceutical Chemistry,
School of Pharmacy, International Medical University, Bukit Jalil,
Kuala Lumpur, Malaysia
[2]Dipartimento di Scienze Chimiche e Farmaceutiche,
Università degli Studi di Trieste, Trieste, Italy
[3]Department of Pharmacy, National University of Singapore,
Singapore, Singapore

ABSTRACT

A_3 adenosine receptor is a G protein-coupled receptor belonging to P1 family of purinergic receptors. It is widely distributed in human organs and tissues with various expression levels. In particular, A_3 adenosine receptor is highly expressed in several immune cells and cancer cell lines. For this reason, its modulation is intensively studied for the involvement in inflammation and cancer. Ligands (agonists and antagonists) presenting high affinity and selectivity for the A_3 adenosine receptor are essential for determining the role of such receptor in these pathophysiological conditions and, eventually, for the development of potential drugs for their treatment. In this review we summarize old and new discoveries on therapeutic applications of the A_3 adenosine receptor in inflammation and cancer, and highlight the most important agonists and antagonists developed for the A_3 adenosine receptor, explicitly those in clinical trials for the treatment of inflammation and/or cancer.

---

[*] Co-first authors.

LIST OF ABBREVIATIONS

AlexaFluor-488	3',6'-diamino-3-oxo-3H-spiro[isobenzofuran-1, 9'-xanthene]-4', 5'-disulfonate
AR	adenosine receptor
BODIPY	boron-dipyrromethene
cAMP	cyclic adenosine monophosphate
CHO	Chinese hamster ovary
Cl-IB-MECA	2-chloro-N6-(3-iodo-benzyl)adenosine-5′-N-methylcarboxamide
CoMFA	Comparative Molecular Field Analysis
DPCPX	8-Cyclopentyl-1, 3-dipropylxanthine
GTPγS	guanosine 5'-O-[γ-thio]triphosphate
HEK-293	human embryonic kidney
HEMADO	2-hexyn-1-yl-N6-methyladenosine
I-ABOPX	3-(3-iodo-4-aminobenzyl)-8-(4-oxyacetate)phenyl-1-propylxanthine
IB-MECA	N6-(4-iodo-benzyl)-5′-N-methylcarboxamide adenosine
IC$_{50}$	half maximal inhibitory concentration
K$_b$	equilibrium dissociation constant of a ligand determined by means of a functional assay
K$_d$	equilibrium dissociation constant of a ligand determined directly in a binding assay using a labelled form of the ligand
K$_i$	equilibrium dissociation constant of a ligand determined in inhibition studies
NECA	5′-N-ethylcarboxamide adenosine
PAMAM	poly(amidoamine)
PENECA	2-phenylethynyl-adenosine-5'-N-ethyluronamide
PET	positron emission tomography
SAR	structure activity relationship

1. INTRODUCTION

There are four main types of human adenosine receptors (hARs) that have been cloned and pharmacologically characterized, namely A$_1$, A$_{2A}$, A$_{2B}$ and A$_3$ ARs [1]. These receptors, which consist of seven transmembrane domains, belong to the large group of G protein-coupled receptors (GPCRs) superfamily that represents a major class of targets for drugs on the market and for those presently in development. In human body, the endogenous purine nucleoside, adenosine, regulates a wide range of physiological responses through interaction with these specific adenosine receptors. They are widely distributed in organs and tissues that render them the potential targets for pharmacological intervention in many pathophysiological conditions [2].

Particularly, there is growing evidence that highlight the importance of A$_3$ adenosine receptors (A$_3$ARs) as a promising therapeutic target and biomarker in inflammation and cancer, given its over-expression in inflammatory and cancer cells as compared to low levels found in normal cells [3]. As such, the need for potent and selective adenosine receptor ligands has become apparent to many scientists. To date, a large number of A$_3$AR agonists and antagonists have been intensively investigated in search of ligands that are able to selectively target the receptor of interest, in order to optimize the desired biological activity and minimize the unwanted side effects.

In this review we give a comprehensive account of discovery, molecular characterization, tissue distribution and signal transduction pathways of the A$_3$AR, as well as its potential role in the inflammatory conditions and cancers. Moreover, relevant therapeutic applications of the A$_3$AR ligands (agonists and antagonists), especially those in clinical trials for the treatment of inflammation or cancer, are also discussed in detail.

1.1. Discovery of A$_3$ Adenosine Receptors

A$_3$ adenosine receptor was initially isolated as an orphan receptor from rat testis in 1991 and designated as tgpcr1 [4]. Thereafter, another identical clone encoding a GPCR was isolated from rat striatum and named as R226 [5]. It was later identified as A$_3$AR, with a nucleotide sequence 99.5% identical to the tgpcr1 [6]. Both clones differ mainly at the C-terminal domain of the receptor, which plays a crucial role in binding to the G protein. Interestingly, similar observation was also found in other GPCR classes (e.g., nicotinic receptors), in which variations at the C-terminus were found between peripheral and central receptors within the same species. Subsequently, homologs of rat striatal A$_3$AR have been identified from sheep and human, in which large interspecies difference in the A$_3$ receptor structure were discovered. There is only 74% sequence homology between the rat A$_3$AR and both sheep and human A$_3$AR, while 85% homology is shown between the sheep and human [2-3, 7]. This has been reflected in considerably different pharmacological profiles of the species homologs, particularly with respect to antagonist binding, which renders characterization of this adenosine receptor difficult.

Among the hARs, hA$_3$AR differs from the highly conserved hA$_1$, hA$_{2A}$ and hA$_{2B}$ receptors. Explicitly, the hA$_3$AR presents a sequence homology of about 61% with hA$_1$AR, 54% with hA$_{2A}$AR and 52% with hA$_{2B}$AR [8]. Contrary to relatively low sequence identity (74%) shared between rat and human A$_3$AR, the cDNA sequences of the other adenosine receptors are highly conserved between rat and human (e.g., human and rat A$_1$ receptors are 89% identical across the open reading frame) [3, 7]. Such species difference in A$_3$AR has led to discrepancy in pharmacological profiles between human and rat, thus hindering the progress towards *in vivo* studies for efficacy and toxicity evaluations, especially for the human A$_3$AR antagonists, in rodent models. The first successful attempt to overcome this limitation was achieved by Yamano and co-workers, who generated a mouse model presenting the A$_3$AR gene with a chimeric human/mouse sequence, which has showed a great correlation between cell biology and animal studies for the human A$_3$AR antagonists [9].

1.2. Molecular Characterization of A_3 Adenosine Receptors

A_3AR has been mapped on human chromosome 1p21-p13 [10] and it is made up of 318 amino acids. The A_3AR gene consists of two exons divided by a single intron of about 2.2 kb [8]. Notably, the upstream sequence contains a few consensus binding sites for a number of transcription factors (e.g., GATA3, which is T-cell specific), suggesting an involvement of this receptor in immune function.

Structurally, the A_3AR is characterized by a polypeptide chain forming seven transmembrane (TM) domains with extracellular N-terminus and cytosolic C-terminus, connected by three intracellular (ICL) and three extracellular loops (ECL) [11]. Sites for post-translational glycosylation have been identified in the extracellular portion, while those for palmitoylation are found at the C-terminal domain. The latter domain also presents a few conserved histidine (His) residues reported to be crucial in recognition and/or modulation of adenosine receptors [12], as well as high density of serine (Ser) and threonine (Thr) residues which could be the potential phosphorylation sites for receptor desensitization and internalization after ligand binding [13 14]. In fact, several studies have described the occurrence of A_3AR desensitization and internalization in some human and rat cancer cells upon treatment with the A_3AR agonists [15]. In addition, an increasing number of studies have reported that GPCRs are arranged in high-ordered molecular structures, of which receptor multimers and other interacting proteins form functional complexes. In the case of the A_3AR, a recent ligand-binding kinetics study conducted by May et al. [16] has identified and quantified co-operative interactions between allosteric and/or orthosteric ligands across the native A_3AR homodimers. Such investigation has provided new insights into the influence of dimerization on the ligand-GPCR interactions. Moreover, a computational prediction of homodimerization of the A_3AR has also been previously illustrated by Jacobson and co-workers [17].

1.3. Biochemical Pathways of A_3 Adenosine Receptors

A_3AR couples to G protein-mediated second messenger pathways through activation of G_i and G_q protein (Figure 1) [13, 18]. It results in G_i protein-mediated inhibition of adenylyl cyclase with a subsequent decrease in cAMP level as well as an increase in G_q protein-mediated phospholipase C activity and calcium ion mobilization [13, 18-19, 20]. Additionally, other secondary pathways have been reported as pertinent to activation of A_3AR; for example, the A_3AR-mediated activation of RhoA with consequent stimulation of phospholipase D (PLD) and protein kinase C (PKC) [21] or the ATP-sensitive potassium channel activation (designated as K_{ATP}) have been reported [22]. Both of the signaling pathways are evidenced to play a role in the cardioprotective function against ischemia/reperfusion (IR) injury [22-23].

On top of that, A_3AR is also related to activation of mitogen-activated protein kinase (MAPKs) [24] or extracellular signal-regulated kinase (ERK1/2) [24-25] through stimulation of Ras, leading to modulation of mitogenesis. The A_3AR-mediated ERK1/2 phosphorylation has been reported in mouse microglia cells, colon carcinoma and glioblastoma [26, 27]. Conversely, A_3AR activation does not stimulate the ERK phosphorylation in the melanoma cells; its stimulation was found to counteract A_{2A}-induced cell death but also to ensure cell survival [28]. In rat cardiomyocytes, the A_3AR-induced ERK1/2 phosphorylation has also been shown to play a role in preconditioning during hypoxia and reoxygenation [29].

Furthermore, the A_3AR is also associated with another biochemical pathway, phosphoinositine 3-kinase (PI3K)/Akt [18]. The activation of A_3AR has been demonstrated to stimulate phosphorylation of Akt in rat cardiomyocytes that results in cardio-protection [30, 31]. On the other hand, the corresponding stimulation of PI3K/Akt by A_3AR activation was shown to trigger inhibition of apoptosis and cause an increase in matrix metalloproteinase-9 (MMP-9) in the glioblastoma cells, resulting in tumor cell proliferation [27, 32]. Moreover, such pathway is also implicated in anti-inflammatory activities mediated by the A_3AR; the activation of A_3AR was shown to suppress tumor necrosis factor (TNF)-α and interleukin (IL)-12 production by inhibiting PI3K/Akt-NF-κB pathway in BV2 microglial cells and monocytes [33, 34, 35].

1.4. Distribution of A₃ Adenosine Receptors

The A_3AR is widely distributed in the organs and tissues. However, there are remarkable differences in expression levels of A_3AR within and between the species. For rat A_3AR, it is largely found in the testis and mast cells, whereas low levels have been detected in other rat tissues [36]. On the other hand, the highest distribution of human A_3AR is found in the lung and liver, while the lowest density has been discovered in the aorta and brain [37, 38].

Through radioligand binding, immunohistochemical and functional studies, the presence of A_3AR protein has been examined in a variety of primary cells, tissues and cell lines [2]. Of note, A_3AR has been found in various primary cells involved in inflammatory conditions. In rat mast cells (RBL-2H3), binding assays have revealed a high density of A_3AR; in fact, various studies have reported the role of A_3AR in rat mast cell degranulation [39, 40]. Recently, A_3AR-stimulated degranulation has been evidenced in the human mast cells [41]. Furthermore, the A_3AR has also been detected in other primary cells engaged in inflammatory responses, such as human eosinophils [42], neutrophils [43, 44], monocytes [45], macrophages [46, 47, 48], dendritic cells [49, 50, 51] and lymphocytes [52]. Besides that, a great variety of cancer cell lines [53, 54, 55, 56, 57] and tissues [58, 59] have shown substantially high expression of this receptor subtype as well, suggesting its potential role as a tumoral marker and target for tumor growth inhibition. More details on the role of A_3AR in inflammation and cancer are provided in the sections 2 & 3.

On the contrary, no direct evidence regarding the presence of A_3AR has been reported in cardiac myocytes to date [60, 61]. Nonetheless, a number of studies have indicated the role of A_3AR on cardioprotection in various models, including isolated cardiomyocytes [62, 63]. Apart from that, low level of A_3AR binding sites has also been observed in the brains of rat, mouse and rabbit; [64] for instances, the expression of this receptor subtype has been found in microglia and astrocytes, the immune cells of the central nervous system [26, 65, 66].

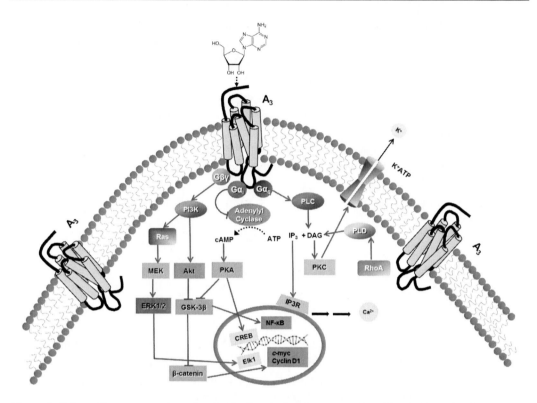

Figure 1. Schematic representation of main biochemical pathways mediated by A₃AR activation.

2. THE ROLE OF A₃ ADENOSINE RECEPTORS IN INFLAMMATION

2.1. Introduction

The fact that all inflammatory cells express ARs is a clear evidence that adenosine has indeed an important signaling role in the pathophysiology of inflammation. An additional proof is that, in case of stress or injury, a massive amount of extracellular adenine nucleotides are converted into adenosine, which then promotes immunosuppressive activities [67, 68]. In that instance, extracellular adenosine is produced from the dephosphorylation of extracellu-lar nucleotides [69] by ectonucleoside triphosphate diphosphohydrolase CD39 (nucleoside triphosphate diphosphohydrolase (NTPDase)) first and 5'-ectonucleotidase CD73 later on regulatory T cells' (Tregs) surface.

Further increase might derive from the suppression of the activity of adenosine kinases (AKs), which prevent the re-phosphorylation of adenosine to adenosine monophosphate (AMP) [70]. Notably, several cell types are sources of these adenine nucleotides, such as platelet and endothelial cells, activated leukocytes & macrophages and T-helper lymphocytes, which are key regulators of the inflammatory response [71, 72, 73, 74, 75]. It is thus not surprising that in the case of inflammation, the extracellular levels of adenosine surge from homeostatic 10-200 nM up to 100 μM [76]. Subsequently, by interacting with cell-surface ARs, adenosine mediates a cascade of intracellular signaling events that vary on the basis of the AR subtype and cell.

Table 1. Inflammatory cells and effects (pro- or anti-inflammatory) mediated by adenosine receptors

Immune cells	Expression of ARs	Effect mediated by A_1AR	Effect mediated by $A_{2A}AR$	Effect mediated by $A_{2B}AR$	Effect mediated by A_3AR
Monocytes and macrophages	All 4 ARs	Pro-inflammatory	Anti-inflammatory	Anti-inflammatory	mainly Anti-inflammatory ($\downarrow$ NADPH oxidase $\downarrow$ ROS, suppression of TNF-α and of IL-12 synthesis)
Neutrophils	All 4 ARs	Pro-inflammatory	Anti-inflammatory	Anti-inflammatory	Both Pro-and Anti-inflammatory ($\downarrow$ degranulation $\downarrow$ cAMP, $\downarrow O_2^-$, $\uparrow\downarrow$ chemotaxis)
Eosinophils	Higher A_3AR mRNA levels	Pro-inflammatory	No evident effect	No evident effect	Anti-inflammatory, but only in human eosinophils
Mast Cells	All ARs apart from A_1AR and debated A_3AR	-	No evident effect	Promotes release of pro-inflammatory mediators	Promotes mast cell degranulation
Lymphocytes	All ARs apart from A_1AR in $CD4^+$ and $CD8^+$ T lymphocytes	Pro-inflammatory	Anti-inflammatory	Anti-inflammatory (decreased IL-2 production)	Pro-inflammatory ($\downarrow$ cAMP, $\downarrow$NF-kB, IL-6, TNF-α, IL-1β)
Dendritic cells (DCs)	Mainly $A_{2A}AR$ in mature DCs	-	Anti-inflammatory, (through stimulation of anti-inflammatory IL-10 production)	-	Ca^{2+} increase
Endothelial cells	Mainly $A_{2A}AR$ and $A_{2B}AR$	Pro-inflammatory	Anti-inflammatory	Anti-inflammatory	Anti-inflammatory $\uparrow$migration

2.2. Immune Cells and Inflammation

Table 1 summarizes the main roles mediated by adenosine receptors on different cells involved in inflammation.

2.2.1. Monocytes and Macrophages

Monocytes and macrophages represent the body's first line of innate immune defense in response to a phatogenic assault. They all express ARs, although their levels vary on the basis of the cells' differentiation and maturation [77, 45] and it seems to be crucial in the resolution of the inflammatory process. In monocytes, A_1ARs are pro-inflammatory (through a rapid increase in the activity of Fcγ receptor [78] and release of Vascular Endothelial Growth Factor (VEGF) [79], while $A_{2A}AR$ are anti-inflammatory (through the suppression of the pro-inflammatory cytokines TNF-α [80] & IL-12, or the stimulation of the anti-inflammatory cytokine IL-10 (also mediated by $A_{2B}AR$) [81, 82, 83, 84, 85, 86]. Conversely, as already mentioned in section 1.3., activation of A_3AR has either no effect [87] or suppresses [33, 35, 34] tumor necrosis factor alpha (TNF-α) and it inhibits the synthesis of IL-12, probably through the phosphatidyl inositol 3-kinase signaling pathway [33, 35, 34, 88].

2.2.2. Neutrophils

Neutrophils are the prevalent leukocytes in the body and they express all the four ARs [76, 89, 90, 91]. Depending on the concentration of adenosine, we assist at different effects: pro-inflammatory at submicromolar concentrations (mediated by A_1AR) and anti-inflammatory, through the activation of $A_{2A}AR$ [which blocks the formation of reactive oxygen species (ROS) [73, 92, 93], endothelium's surface proteins [94, 95] and pro-inflammatory cytokines like TNF-α, platelet activating factor (PAF) [96], leukotriene LTB4] [97, 98, 99, 100, 101, 102, 103] and $A_{2B}AR$ [which prevents the release of VEGF] [104].

Both pro- and anti-inflammatory effects have been ascribed to the activation of A_3AR: on one side, extracellular adenosine concentrations < 1μM have been associated with neutrophils' recruitment upon chemoattractant molecule release. On the other hand, A_3AR activation has shown to inhibit degranulation and oxidative stress [43, 44, 105].

2.2.3. Eosinophils

Eosinophils are involved in allergic reactions and asthma, whereby they infiltrate the inflamed airway and release inflammatory mediators (e.g., ROS, leukotrienes etc.). Interestingly, while A_1AR activation exacerbates superoxide release, A_3ARs (whose mRNA was observed to be overexpressed in patients with airway inflammation),[106] inhibit O_2^- release [107], increase intracellular Ca^{2+} [107] and inhibit PAF-induced chemotaxis [106, 108], although only in human cells.

2.2.4. Mast Cells

Similarly to eosinophils, mast cells are involved in allergic reactions and asthma. Adenosine has an influence on both mast cell degranulation and mediators release for both immediate and chronic effects in the case of inflamed airway. A_3AR and $A_{2B}AR$ seem to play a pivotal role, whereby A_3AR mediates mast cell degranulation (through PI3K activation and enhanced intracellular Ca^{2+} levels) [109, 110], while A$_{2B}$AR promotes release of pro-inflammatory mediators such as IL-4, IL-8 and IL-13 [111, 112, 113].

2.2.5. Lymphocytes

Similar to neutrophils, the effects on different lymphocytes depend on the adenosine concentrations: at low concentrations (1-100 nM) A$_1$AR activity prevails, thus inhibiting cAMP production, while at high levels of adenosine (100 nM-100 μM) cAMP production surges upon A$_{2A}$AR activation [89, 114]. More precisely, CD4$^+$ and CD8$^+$ T lymphocytes express all ARs apart from A$_1$AR subtype [115, 116, 117, 118, 119, 52, 120]. A$_{2A}$AR activation in CD4$^+$ T lymphocytes mediates anti-inflammatory effects by inhibiting T-cell receptor (TCR)-mediated production of IFN-γ, TNF-α and IL-4, thus limiting both T-cell activation and also macrophage activation in inflamed tissues [121] Conversely, pro-inflammatory effects have been attributed to both A$_1$AR and A$_3$AR subtypes [122].

In B lymphocytes, adenosine has shown to inhibit the nuclear factor kappa B (NF-kB) pathway through an increased level of cAMP and activation of protein kinase A.

Finally, in activated natural killer (NK) cells, adenosine blocks the production of cytokines and chemokines; [123, 124] more precisely, A$_{2A}$AR decreases while A$_1$AR increases NK cell activity [125].

2.2.6. Dendritic Cells

Dendritic cells (DCs) are specialized antigen presenting cells (APCs) that migrate to sites of injury, process antigens and activate naïve T cells [126, 127]. After maturation (upon exposure to pathogens or pro-inflammatory molecules (e.g., TNF-α, IL-1 and IL-6) [126], they release TNF-α, IL-10 and IL-12, the last of which is highly involved in the differentiation of T cells into Th 1 phenotype. Mature DCs express mainly A$_{2A}$AR [49, 128] and their activation is responsible for the increase in adenylate cyclase's activity (with subsequent increased levels of cAMP and p42/p44 MAPK phosphorylation), inhibition of IL-12 production and stimulation of IL-10 production [126, 128].

2.2.7. Endothelial Cells

In case of inflammation, vascular endothelium increases permeability to allow the newly recruited leukocytes to permeate into the site of damage. On this regards, ARs are expressed heterogeneously (with the highest abundance of A$_{2A}$AR and A$_{2B}$AR subtypes) [129, 130, 131, 132, 133] on these cells and they mediate both anti-inflammatory and pro-inflammatory effects. More precisely, A$_{2A}$AR activation inhibits the expression of vascular cell adhesion molecule-1 (VCAM-1) [134] and tissue factor [130]. Moreover, together with A$_{2B}$AR, it also alleviates the progression of inflammation by decreasing the permeability to leukocytes. Conversely, A$_1$AR is involved in release of cytotoxic molecules that increase the endothelium's permeability [135].

2.3. Adenosine Receptors Involved in Inflammation

All four ARs are expressed on monocytes and macrophages, although their expression increases upon inflammatory spur [77, 45]. It seems that this drastic change is crucial to terminate the inflammatory process. However, not all the ARs are associated with anti-inflammatory effects.

2.3.1. A_1AR in inflammation

Indeed, activation of A_1AR is responsible for pro-inflammatory effects through the induction of VEGF release from monocytes, neutrophil chemotaxis, Fcγ receptor-mediated phagocytosis and superoxide (O_2-) generation [78, 136]. This exacerbation of inflammation has been confirmed *in vivo* in several models including ischemia-reperfusion injury of lungs [137], heart [138, 139, 140] and liver [141, 142] as well as pancreatitis [143] and asthma [144, 145]. Adenosine deaminase (ADA, which is responsible for the biotransformation of the endogenous modular adenosine into its deaminated form, i.e., inosine)/ A_1AR double-knockout mice developed pulmonary inflammation, characterized by elevated levels of pro-inflammatory cytokines (mainly IL-3 and IL-4) and chemokines (e.g., eotaxin 2 and thymus- and activation-regulated chemokine). Conversely, a protective role by A_1AR has been observed in renal ischemia-reperfusion model [146], possibly due to the phosphorylation of ERK MAPK and Akt, as well as of heat shock protein (HSP) 27 [147, 148].

2.3.2. $A_{2A}AR$ in inflammation

$A_{2A}AR$ has shown to be the major AR mediating the anti-inflammatory effects of adenosine [149], by inhibiting O_2- formation from neutrophils [73] and limiting the production of inflammatory species including IL-12, TNF-α and IFNγ [82, 150] from monocytes [82], dendritic [151] and T cells [121]. In addition, activation of $A_{2A}AR$ promotes wound healing [152] and prevents oxidative surge [73] and neutrophil migration [136]. Several animal models of inflammatory bowel disease (IBD) [153], ischemic liver damage [154], renal injury [155], myocardial injury [156, 157], lung transplantation [158] and spinal cord injury [159] have confirmed the beneficial role of $A_{2A}AR$ in tissues and organs associated with acute inflammation and hypoxia. More precisely, in the last reported three disease models, the anti-inflammatory and tissue-protective effects of $A_{2A}AR$ agonists have been ascribed to the $A_{2A}AR$ expression on bone marrow-derived cells (specifically CD1d-activated natural killer NK T cells), while for the IBD model Tregs were shown to be crucial [153]. Finally, $A_{2A}AR$ agonists, although with some contradicting reports [160], have demonstrated to be promising, anti-asthmatic agents on the basis of the $A_{2A}AR$-mediated decreased pulmonary inflammation, mucus secretion and alveolar airway destruction observed in an allergic lung inflammatory model [161].

However, activation of $A_{2A}AR$, if useful for many diseases where inflammation is involved, might become detrimental in other conditions, where for example $A_{2A}AR$-mediated immunosuppressive activities protect certain tumors from the body's effort to eliminate them [162]. As such, the combination of antitumor T cells with A_{2A} gene deletion might represent a promising strategy for cancer immunotherapy.

2.3.3. $A_{2B}AR$ in inflammation

As regards $A_{2B}AR$, this subtype has a low affinity for adenosine, therefore its expression is mainly induced when adenosine concentrations surge, namely in hypoxic and inflammatory conditions [163, 164]. This aspect, unique among the ARs, might suggest that $A_{2B}AR$ activation has an important role especially in pathological conditions [76]. Indeed, the most established anti-inflammatory effect attributed to $A_{2B}AR$ activation is its ability, derived from its interaction with adenylate cyclase and correspondent increase of cAMP levels, to inhibit macrophage and monocyte functions, including the blockage of the release of pro-inflammatory cytokines (IL-1β and TNF-α) from monocytes or macrophages and the increased production of IL-10 from macrophages.[86]. Despite these anti-inflammatory effects, there have been several reports indicating that $A_{2B}AR$ mediates pro-inflammatory effects as well [165, 113, 166], probably through both G_s and G_q pathways [167, 168] These pro-inflammatory activities were confirmed in a few animal models of IBD (where IL-6 was released upon activation of $A_{2B}AR$) [168] and especially in the lung, suggesting a beneficial use of $A_{2B}AR$ antagonists in the treatment of asthma, pulmonary fibrosis and chronic obstructive pulmonary disease (COPD).

2.3.4. A₃AR in Inflammation

It has been shown that A_3AR is able to decrease the production of TNF-α in various macrophage cell lines [80, 48, 169, 170]. In human neutrophils, this receptor, together with the $A_{2A}AR$ subtype, mediates the reduction of superoxide formation [43, 44]. Besides this anti-inflammatory effect, A_3AR favours the migration of neutrophils at the site of inflammation, thus promoting an additional pro-inflammatory effect (Figure 2) [171].

Pro-inflammatory effects have been also attributed to A_3AR expressed on mast cells, where activation of this receptor increased intracellular levels of Ca^{2+} through the coupling of G_i to PI3K [110], with consequent mast cell degranulation (although in some studies mast cell degranulation was ascribed to $A_{2B}AR$ rather than A_3AR) [172]. An additional mechanism seems to involve protein kinase B phosphorylation [173] promoted by A_3AR activation, which in turn inhibits apoptosis and aggravates inflammation.

Besides mast cells, A_3AR plays a key role in eosinophils, where its activation suppressed eosinophil chemotaxis, degranulation and O_2- production [107] in *ex vivo* studies. It is worth noting that A_3AR's influence on these eosinophils is not a direct effect, and it is neither mediated by cytokines nor chemokines (which are documented to be responsible for eosinophils recruitment); conversely, this process seems to involve other mediators such as adhesion molecules, proteases and/or extracellular matrix proteins [174]. Controversial studies suggested that this receptor seems to influence eosinophil activation and degranulation to different extents [175, 176].

Overall, it still remains unclear how cells expressing A_3AR are influencing each other, so that we observe either pro- or anti-inflammatory effects. More *in vivo* experiments in animal models of inflammation and in humans are necessary before any conclusion can be drawn on the role of A_3AR in inflammation.

2.4. A₃AR in Inflammation-Related Diseases

The anti-inflammatory effects mediated by A_3AR in several pathological conditions rely on the inhibition of NF-κB signaling pathway, which causes the inhibition of downstream pro-inflammatory cytokine expression [177], concomitant decrease in TNF-α, inhibition of macrophage inflammatory proteins (MIPs-1α, MIP-2), and receptor activator of NF-κB ligand (RANKL), finally resulting in apoptosis of inflammatory cells [178, 179, 180]. In addition, a direct antiproliferative effect towards autoreactive T cells upon A_3AR stimulation has been observed [181].

2.4.1. Asthma and Chronic Obstructive Pulmonary Disease (COPD)

Asthma is a disease affecting the lungs, whereby bronchial hyperresponsiveness (BHR) and inflammation are key features. Several triggers have been identified to cause this BHR, including migration and activation of inflammatory cells (e.g., DCs, eosinophils and T lymphocytes) [182, 183, 184, 185, 186], altered epithelial cell function [187] and altered smooth muscle function [188, 189].

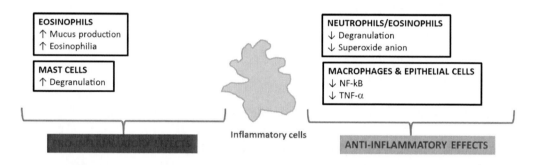

Figure 2. A_3AR influencing inflammatory cells.

Asthmatic people bronchoconstrict upon exposure to both physiological stimuli (e.g., distilled water, cold air, exercise etc.) and chemical substances including adenosine, which are all innocuous substances for non-diseased individuals and are thus are referred as "indirect-acting stimuli." With regards to adenosine, several reports have confirmed the involvement of this purine nucleoside in the pathogenic profile of asthma, including (but not limited to) 1) dose-dependent bronchoconstriction observed in asthmatic exposed to adenosine; 2) release of bronchoconstrictive molecules in patients challenged with an adenosine precursor (AMP); [190] 3) elevated adenosine levels in exhaled breath condensate in asthmatic individuals [191].

In fact adenosine causes bronchoconstriction in airways by directly acting on ARs in bronchial smooth muscle cells or indirectly, by promoting the liberation of inflammatory mediators from mast cells or even by affecting afferent sensory nerves [192, 193, 194, 195] Adenosine-mediated inflammation is not confined within the lung, but it also extend to the systemic circulation, as testified by an increase in 9α, 11β-prostaglandin F2 levels in plasma after adenosine challenge in asthmatics [196].

Despite this evidence, the relevance of A_3AR in the pathophysiology of asthma or of poor airflow as in COPD [197] is highly controversial, mainly due to remarkable species differences. In mice, rats and guinea pigs, A_3AR activation by adenosine induces bronchoconstriction [198], mast cell degranulation, airway inflammation and increase mucus secretion [174], suggesting a promising treatment of asthma with A_3AR antagonists (e.g., KF-26777 under preclinical investigation as anti-asthmatic agent-see Section 5 on A_3AR antagonists). In humans instead, mast cell degranulation is ascribed mainly to $A_{2B}AR$ [111, 172, 112] and A_3AR mediates anti-inflammatory effects, blocking cytokine release from monocytes, as well as chemotaxis and degranulation of eosinophils [107, 175], thus implying that A_3AR agonists should be chosen as therapeutic intervention to treat these conditions.

Overall, it seems that a hybrid agent, for example the one combining both A$_{2B}$AR and A$_3$AR antagonism [199], might represent a promising option, but further studies are required to solve the role of this still-enigmatic receptor in asthma and COPD.

2.4.2. Injury upon Ischemia and Reperfusion

Ischemia is a restriction in blood supply to a certain tissue, with the concomitant shortage of oxygen carrying capacity (i.e., hypoxia) and glucose needed to keep the tissue alive. Ischemic injury increases inflammation, causing the recruitment of circulating polymorphonuclear leukocytes. Up to a certain point, this phenomenon is reversible if blood flow and oxygen supply are restored; however, in some instances the restoration of blood flow may increase local inflammatory cell infiltration, generate oxygen-derived free radicals and exacerbate injury, so-called reperfusion injury. In this context, A$_3$ARs have confirmed a protective role *in vivo* in case of lung injury after ischemia and reperfusion [178, 200], attributable to the up-regulation of phosphorylated ERK [178] opening of ATP-sensitive potassium (K$_{ATP}$) channels and NOS-independent pathways [201], suggesting a promising use of A$_3$AR agonists in inflammatory diseases.

However, in renal ischemia reperfusion injury [202, 203] A$_3$AR worsened renal dysfunction [204, 203] and A$_3$AR antagonists ameliorated the situation. This was also the case of ocular ischemia [205, 206], whereby nucleoside-derived A$_3$AR antagonists lowered mouse intraocular pressure and were able to act across species (i.e., they suggested to be efficacious in multiple animal models).

2.4.3. Inflammatory Bowel Disease (IBD) and Colitis

IBD is characterized by local tissue hypoxia and increased levels of pro-inflammatory cytokines [207]. In this instance, A$_3$AR (and also A$_1$AR and A$_{2B}$AR) show altered expressions [208, 209]. Recently, it was demonstrated that A$_3$AR is expressed in human colonic epithelial cells and, once activated, it mediates an anti-inflammatory effect, through the mechanism described before. These results suggest that A$_3$AR activation may be a potential treatment for abdominal inflammatory diseases such as IBD and colitis or septic peritonis [210].

On line with this, other investigations showed decreased inflammation and higher survival upon A$_3$AR activation in two murine models of colitis [211]. However, this was in contrast with a recent finding on dextran sodium sulfate-induced colitis, where the authors showed a protective effect in functional A$_3$AR $^{-/-}$ knockout mice, thereby suggesting a new hypothesis that A$_3$AR activation does contribute to the disease progression of colitis [212].

2.4.4. Rheumatoid Arthritis (RA)

In the case of rheumatoid arthritis, activation of A$_3$AR could provide protective effects *via* the suppression of pro-inflammatory cytokine secretion through PI3K NF-kB pathway [57] or the inhibition of MIP-1α and TNF-α production [213]. More precisely, A$_3$AR activation down-regulates PI3K, PKB/Akt, I$_\kappa$B kinase (IKK) and inhibitor of $_\kappa$B (I$_\kappa$B), whereby this de-regulation of the NF-kB signaling pathway results in apoptosis of inflammatory cells and inhibition of TNF-α [213, 214, 179, 180]. Interestingly, increased expression of A$_3$AR has been found in the peripheral blood mononuclear cells (PBMCs) of arthritic animals [180, 214, 179] and also in patients with colorectal cancer [52] (see Section

3 for more details on A$_3$AR in cancer), indicating that indeed A$_3$AR may represent a therapeutic target for both inflammation and cancer. Due to this overexpression of A$_3$AR on PBMCs, it is not surprising that the co-administration of an A$_3$AR selective agonist IB-MECA and one of the most used therapeutic agents in RA (i.e., methotrexate, MTX) resulted in additive effects in arthritis animal models [215]. In fact, in the body MTX is converted into polyglutamates, which are known to protect adenosine from degradation, thus promoting drug accumulation in the extracellular fluid [216, 217, 218]. The importance of A$_3$AR is therefore not just in mediating the increased therapeutic efficacy of MTX but, on the basis of its expression, also as a predictive biomarker [219] or an indicator for disease progression in RA.

2.4.5. Eye inflammation

Modulation of A$_3$AR has been also explored for the treatment of inflammatory ophthalmic diseases such as dry eye and uveoretinitis [220]. Dry eye disease is an inflammation of the eye and it is associated with excessive production of proinflammatory cytokines [221, 222]. These inflammatory mediators induce the maturation of APCs and their migration to draining lymphoid tissues. These APCs prime naïve T cells in the lymphoid tissues, causing the expansion of autoreactive CD4$^+$ helper T cell (TH) subtype 1 and T$_H$17 cell subtypes. These TH cells subsequently infiltrate the ocular surface, where they secrete additional proinflammatory cytokines [223]. The stimulation of A$_3$AR in two clinical trials has shown to provide significant improvement in the prognosis of dry eye probably through an A$_3$AR-mediated interaction on inflammatory cells [224], although additional studies on reduction of inflammation are required to fully confirm this aspect.

2.4.6. Skin Inflammation

Psoriasis is an immune-mediated systemic itchy condition characterized by skin lesions such as scaly patches, and pklaques [225]. In this skin condition, dendritic cells produce interleukin (IL)-12 and IL-23, involved in TH1 and TH17 lymphocyte differentiation, respectively. IL-1, secreted by activated macrophages, is crucial mediator of the inflammatory response. Tumour necrosis factor (TNF)-α, IL-17, IL-22 and IL-26 stimulate keratinocyte release of adhesion molecules, cytokines, and chemokines, which, further attract neutrophils and T lymphocytes, thus leading to exacerbation of inflammation [226]. Adenosine has been reported to play an important role in immunity and skin inflammation [227], and in particular the A$_{2A}$ adenosine receptor subtype has shown the ability to modulate inflammatory processes besides promoting wound healing. Moreoevr, Arasa and collaborators demonstrated that the topical application of a selective A$_{2A}$ agonist, CGS 21680, to mouse skin reduced epidermal hyperplasia as well as skin inflammation, similarly to topical corticoids, without side effects like skin atrophy [228].

As regards the A$_3$ receptor subtype, it has been shown to be over-expressed in patients with psoriasis, suggesting its role in the treatment of skin diseases. CF101 (IB-MECA) is an A$_3$AR agonist that downregulates the nuclear factor-κB signalling pathway. It is currently in Phase III clinical trials (Can-Fite BioPharma) [226].

2.5. Summary on Inflammation

Extensive research into the implication of ARs' modulation has opened new opportunities for adenosine-based therapeutic intervention. Taken together, *in vitro* experiments in inflammatory cells and *in vivo* studies in animal models seem to suggest that ARs are important targets in inflammation; more precisely, A_1AR antagonists might be beneficial as anti-inflammatory agents, as demonstrated by several ongoing phase I/II/III clinical studies for chronic congestive heart failure with renal impairment (e.g., http://www.clinicaltrials.gov) [229, 230, 231]. $A_{2A}AR$ is able to modulate inflammatory processes besides promoting wound healing [227].

Finally, CF101 was found to display a protective role in several mouse models of inflammatory diseases, suggesting that A_3AR agonists might represent a novel, promising family of orally bioavailable drugs in the treatment of inflammatory diseases [232].

3. A₃ ADENOSINE RECEPTOR AND CANCER

3.1. Introduction

A_3AR is a therapeutic target that has only been in the field of cancer therapy for 14 years. The first observation of its therapeutic effect was by Fishman P. et al. in 2001. The activation of A_3AR was first observed to exert a therapeutic effect *via* increasing the number of cells in the G_0/G_1 phase and decreasing the telomeric signal, inhibiting tumour cell growth and proliferation. It was also observed to cause the expression of the granulocyte-colony-stimulating factor, stimulating the murine bone marrow cell proliferation [233]. With the confirmation that the activation of A_3ARs could modulate the cell growth and initiate cytokines' expression and that the A_3ARs agonists could function as anticancer agents, since 2001 there has been a surging interest in tuning research on A_3ARs to 1) further understand their role in cancer and the differential expression of A_3ARs in tumour cells *versus* normal cells; 2) evaluate the possible effects of activation and inactivation of A_3ARs on tumour proliferation and metastasis.

As mentioned in Section 1, A_3ARs are observed to be highly overexpressed in tumour cells as compared to normal cells [234]. A study by Madi et al. in 2004 has shown that the intensity of the A_3ARs, with a molecular weight of 39kDa, in the normal cells in both the colon and breast tissues are almost non-existent. However, the level of A_3ARs in the tumour cells of colon carcinoma and breast carcinoma are significantly higher as compared to normal cells. Hence, there is a widespread interest in exploiting A_3ARs, both as a potential therapeutic target as well as a cancer biomarker [58].

3.2. A₃ Adenosine Receptor and Cancer Signaling Pathways

A summary of the main signaling pathways involving A_3AR is depicted in Table 2.

Table 2. Involvement of A₃AR in different cancer signaling pathways

Cancer Signaling Pathways	References
ERK1/2 pathway	[235, 236. 237, 238, 239, 240, 241, 242, 243]
Wnt signaling pathway	[34, 35, 59, 244, 245, 246, 247, 248]
cAMP	[249, 250, 251]
p53	[238, 252, 253, 254]
Ang-2	[255, 256]

The activation of A_3AR would result in a down-regulation of adenylate cyclase, causing a decrease in the formation of cAMP. The reduction in cAMP would result in a downregulation of protein kinase A catalytic subunit (PKA_c) and of NF-κB of activated B cells. As shown in Figure 3, the upregulation of the nuclear factor of kappa light polypeptide gene enhancer in B-cells inhibitor (IκB) kinase, which phosphorylate the IκB of IκB-p50-p65-p complex, prevents the release of the p50-p65 heterodimer, the NF-κB complex [234]. The reduced level of the NF-κB complex prevents the binding and hence, the activation of the kappa B (κB) site of the gene, inhibiting the transcription and translation of genes that would promote inflammation. Cellular inflammation near the tumour cell regions would ultimately result in improved survival and proliferation of both the tumour cells and endogenous normal cells surrounding the tumour. Inflammatory cells near the sites of the tumour would promote further growth of the tumour rather than cause cell death *via* apoptosis. This is due to the ability of the tumour cells to recruit the inflammatory cells to provide a supply of growth factors and thus enhance their survival and proliferation; indeed, one of the hallmarks of cancer is the acquired capability to be self-sufficient in growth signals [257]. In addition, NF-κB was shown to play an important function in the regulation of the cell cycle *via* modulating the cyclin D1 expression. NF-κB was shown to cause an increase in the cyclin D1 expression in the G1 phase of the cell cycle [258]. A high level of cyclin D1 during G1 phase is necessary to initiate the DNA synthesis in the cell prior to S phase of cell mitosis [259]. Hence, by down-regulating the activity of NF-κb in the tumour cells, it would in principle prevent their proliferation.

In addition, the activation of $A_{3A}ARs$ would result in the down-regulation of the wnt signaling pathway, also known as the phosphoinositide 3-kinase-protein kinase B (PKB/Akt) pathway. It occurs *via* the inhibition of the formation of cAMP. The low cAMP level prevents the formation of the receptor complex involving Frizzled family receptor and a few co-receptors. This results in the reduction of the activation of the protein complexes containing GSK3β, β-catenin and other proteins. A reduction in the phosphorylation of GSK3β prevents the phosphorylation of the β-catechin, which would allow it to be removed from the cytoplasm *via* ubiquitination and degradation by the proteasome-ubiquitin pathway. This prevents the accumulation and translocation of the phosphorylated β-catechin to the nucleus, which then results in the down-regulation on the level of cyclin D1 and c-Myc.

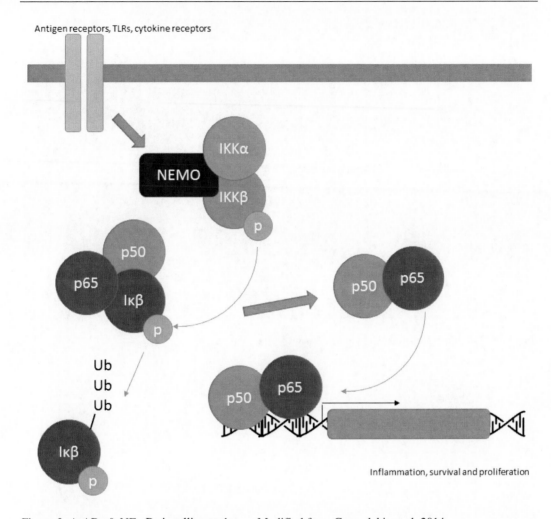

Figure 3. A₃ARs & NF-κB signalling pathway. Modified from Gerondakis et al. 2014.

Although the protein c-Myc is short-lived, c-Myc is an important primary oncogene (Figure 4). It is the "master regulator" that drives cell proliferation by stimulating glycolysis as well as the expression of a broad spectrum of metabolic enzymes. C-Myc is also involved in stimulating the mitochondrial biogenesis, increasing the histone acetylation and fatty acid biosynthesis in highly proliferative cells. c-Myc regulates the glutamate expression providing energy to the cells for both growth and proliferation. However, the use of c-Myc as a therapeutic target proves to be a challenging issue as it undergoes several modifications every few years *via* adaptation to the environment (mutation) upon prolonged exposure to the therapeutic agent during cancer therapy [260].

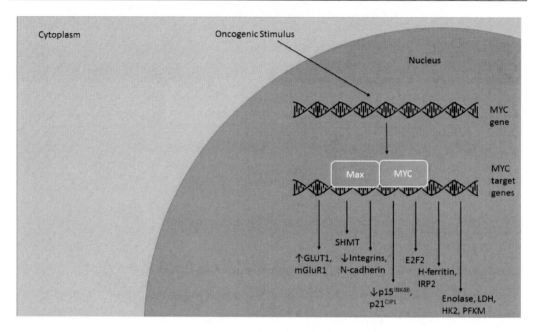

Figure 4. Role of c-Myc in cancer. Modified from Miller et al. 2012.

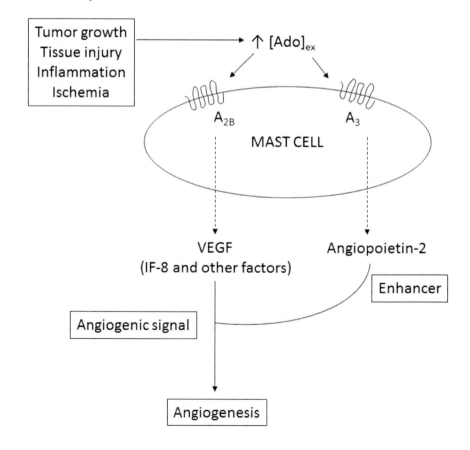

Figure 5. Effects of activation of both A_{2B}ARs and A_3ARs receptors on angiogenesis. Modified from Feoktistov et al. 2003.

However, it is also worth to note that the activation of A$_3$ARs also induces the expression of angiopoietin-2 (Figure 5). This promotes neo-vascularization in angiogenesis of tumour cells if the A$_{2B}$ARs are also activated, due to VEGF secretion. If the A$_{2B}$ARs are not activated, the induced expression of angiopoietin-2 would result in an opposite effect, i.e., on the inhibition of the endothelial cell-specific receptor tyrosine kinase Tie2 (TEK) and destabilization of the blood vessels, preventing angiogenesis.[255] In the case of both the presence of A$_{2B}$ARs and A$_3$ARs, the use of A$_3$AR antagonists would be necessary to prevent angiogenesis and hence, the metastasis of tumour cells.

This would pose a very challenging issue as the A$_3$AR ligands have to be very A$_3$-selective, otherwise they could potentially interact with both A$_{2B}$ARs and A$_3$ARs simultaneously, which would result in the promotion of tumour cell proliferation and metastasis instead of the desired outcome of tumour growth inhibition.

3.3. A$_3$ Adenosine Receptor *versus* Other Adenosine G Protein-Coupled Receptors in Cancer

Both the A$_3$AR and the other adenosine GPCRs had been observed to be upregulated in various tumour cells [261]. More precisely, the A$_1$ARs are overexpressed in the microglia of brain tumour cells as compared to the microglia in normal brain cells. Deficiency of A$_1$ARs in the microglia cells of animal model is observed to result in an accumulation of microglia cells at and around the tumours, as well as cause significant proliferation of glioblastoma. Similarly, human glioblastoma samples were observed to express A$_1$ARs in both microglial as well as tumour cells. Hence, A$_1$ARs agonists are capable of curbing the glioblastoma progression based on observations made on organotypical brain splice cultures [262].

The activation of A$_{2A}$ARs enhances the expression of CD73, which significantly increases the metastatic property of tumour cells. This is achieved *via* the suppression of antitumor immune response, the NK cell function. Therefore, it is suggested that A$_{2A}$AR antagonists would reduce the metastasis of CD73$^+$ tumours *via* the enhancement of the immunoresponse in cancer therapy [263]. In addition, the A$_{2A}$AR in the pulmonary endothelial cells plays a significant role in angiogenesis particularly in human lung cancer. Its gene promoter is revealed to carry a hypoxia-responsive element (HRE) and its activation would result in an increase in cell proliferation, cell migration and tube formation [264]. Therefore, both hypoxia and HIF-2α are possible therapeutic targets since they are responsible for modulating A$_{2A}$AR's activation. HIF-2α is observed to preferentially bind at HRE in the Epo-3' enhancer in the native state of the Epo *locus*. Epo is dominantly regulated by HIF-2α. Epo is a pro-survival growth factor that is capable of inducing erythropoiesis. Epo as a pro-survival growth factor would enhance the viability of tumour cells in a stressed environment, thus the inhibition of the docking of HIF-2α *via* activation of A$_{2A}$ARs would prevent tumour cell viability [265].

The activation of A$_{2B}$ARs *via* CD73-derived adenosine results in the suppression of the prenylation of the small guanosine triphosphate (GTPase) RAS-related protein 1 (RAP1). RAP1 is involved in maintaining functional cell adherent junctions which, upon suppression, results in loss of cell adhesion and significant enhancement of the metastatic property of tumour cells [266]. As mentioned in Section 3.2, A$_{2B}$AR activation promotes angiogenesis when it is co-activated with A$_3$ARs in the human mast cells *via* the paracrine mechanism. The activation of $A_{2B}ARs$ induces the expression of interleukin-8 (IL-8), which stimulates angiogenesis in various solid tumours, and VEGF, another potent angiogenic factor. The activation of A_3ARs induces the expression of angiopoietin-2, which promotes neo-vascularization in conjunction with VEGF secretion. The human mast cells are observed to tend to concentrate around the blood vessels during inflammation and neoplastic foci and this accumulation is significant in the proximity of the tumour cells before the occurrence of tumour-associated angiogenesis. The activation of these human mast cells by adenosine triggers the synthesis and release of the abovementioned angiogenic factors from the mast cells, thus exacerbating angiogenesis [255]. Overall, research on adenosine receptors, investigating the possible therapeutic effects of the various adenosine receptors' antagonists as well as agonists, has confirmed that $A_{3A}ARs$ agonists are likely to function effectively as chemotherapeutic agents (more details on $A_{3A}ARs$ agonists are in Section 4) [7].

Other adenosine receptors are present in various tissues and cells, which make the selective targeting of adenosine receptors in the tumour cells difficult [267]. Treatment targeting other adenosine receptors would increase the risk of possible side and adverse effects. This would account for the surging interest in the study of A_3AR and its role in cancer therapy.

3.4. A_3 Adenosine Receptor and Melanoma

Many research studies of A_3AR and their therapeutic effect on cancer are focused on a type of skin cancer called melanoma. The commonly used cell line for detecting the effect of A_3AR activator and antagonist on melanoma is the A375 melanoma cell line. The A375 melanoma cell line is often used because these cells have been found to highly express A_3ARs. The level of A_3ARs in the melanoma cells allows A_3ARs to act as biomarker, as A_3ARs are not expressed in the normal skin cells. Moreover, it was reported that the activation of A_3ARs with an A_3AR agonist, Cl-IB-MECA, is capable of suppressing the proliferation of melanoma cells *via* the deregulation of the wnt signaling pathway by decreasing the PKA level, a downstream cAMP effector, as well as by deregulating the PKB/Akt pathway. The downstream effects of the deregulation, as previously described, result in the inhibition of the proliferation of melanoma cells [15, 268].

This receptor has also been observed to modulate the level of hypoxia-Inducible Factor-1α (HIF-1α), which is elevated during hypoxia condition. HIF-1α is a key regulator of genes of growth factors that are necessary for tumour growth. A study on the effect of A_3ARs on HIF-1α concluded that the stimulation of A_3ARs would activate the p44/p42 and p38 mitogen-activated protein kinases, which increased the level of HIF-1α. The up-regulation of HIF-1α induces the expression of Ang-2, which would induce angiogenesis in the presence of VEGF [256]. Hence, in the case of advanced stage cancer, the use of A_3AR antagonists proves to be a novel and promising therapeutic agent in cancer therapy, as A_3AR antagonists are capable of preventing the up-regulated expression of Ang-2, which would otherwise accelerate the process of angiogenesis.

A_3AR activation would also activate the ERK1/2 MAP kinases, which would increase the level of matrix metalloproteinases (MMPs) such as MMP-1, MMP-2 and MMP-9, which would increase the capability of tumour cells to invade other parts of the body *via* metastasis

[269]. These interesting findings justify the growing interest on the effect of A$_3$AR antagonists on metastatic cancer.

3.5. A$_3$ Adenosine Receptor and Carcinoma

Carcinoma is the other more studied cancer to investigate A$_3$AR's effect on tumour cell growth. It has been reported that the activation of A$_3$ARs could also inhibit colon, breast and prostrate carcinoma growth and liver metastasis *via* the above mentioned de-regulation of the wnt and NF-κb signaling pathways [248]. The activation of A$_3$ARs has also been observed to result in apoptosis of cancer cells. This conclusion was made based on the effect of 2-Cl-IB-MECA on Lu-85 human lung cancer cells. It is postulated that the pathway through which the activation of A$_3$ARs would cause apoptosis is *via* the up-regulated expression of p53 and Noxa mRNAs. Both p53 and Noxa mRNAs are heavily involved in inducing the apoptosis of tumour cells. The study on 2-Cl-IB-MECA also confirmed that capase-3 and capase-9 are enhanced upon activation of A$_3$ARs. Both capase-3 and capase-9 are proteins peptidase involved in the apoptosis process [252].

The activation of A$_3$ARs is also observed to result in the inhibition of the nicotinamide adenine dinucleotide phosphate (NADPH) oxidase activity, which is responsible for the formation of reactive oxygen species (ROS) that have shown to exacerbate the growth of prostate cancer. The NADPH oxidase subunits involved are gp91^{phox} and NOX5, based on studies conducted on androgen-dependent PC3 and androgen-independent DU145 prostate cancer cell lines. The ROS are postulated to mediate the mitogenic signaling and regulate the actions of transcription factors, such as activator protein-1 and NF-κB and protein kinases, such as PKc and ERK1/2 MAP kinases. The constitutive activation of ERK1/2 MAP kinases would promote tumour metastasis and cell proliferation. The level of NADPH has been observed to be high in tumour cancer. The agonist-activated A$_3$ARs have been reported to decrease the PKA-mediated stimulation of ERK1/2, reduce the level of membrane-bound p47^{phox} expression, which ultimately results in a decrease in the level of ROS generation in the tumour cells [249].

The activation of A$_3$ARs in prostate carcinoma has also been reported to induce the inhibition of P47^{phox} *via* the inhibition of ERK1/2 MAP kinase activity [270]. This is achieved *via* the cAMP/PKA signaling pathway. P47^{phox} is also involved in the ROS production, which would promote tumour growth.

There is, however, a recent study that claims that the effect of the A$_3$AR agonist on the inhibition of the proliferation of human tyroid carcinoma is not due to the activation of the A$_3$ARs. This was demonstrated by the inability to inhibit the antiproliferative effect of the agonist with the use of an antagonist [271]. The use of other adenosine receptors antagonists, as well as the nucleoside transport inhibitors, were similarly incapable of inhibiting the effect of the agonist. Hence, it remains elusive on whether the activation of A$_3$ARs is applicable to all tumoural cells and tissues, despite the high expression of this receptor as compared to normal cells [271].

3.6. A₃ Adenosine Receptor and Leukemia

Another immunohistochemical study of the human tumour junket cell line showed that also in the case of leukemia there are significant levels of A₃ARs, comparable to those of the A375 melanoma cell line used in other studies [272]. Nevertheless, as of now, there is insufficient investigation on the activation of A₃ adenosine receptor on leukemia to draw any insightful conclusion.

3.7. Final Overview of A₃AR in Cancer

Above is reported a figure (Figure 6) that summarizes all the different cancer signaling pathways that are observed in the various tumour cells, with many tumour cells having overlapping signaling pathways.

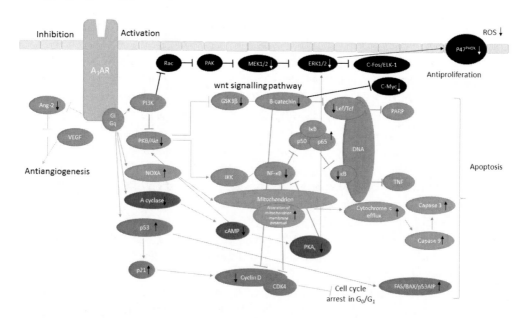

Figure 6. Different signaling pathway involved in various tumour cells.

Based on the above figure, A₃AR modulation seems to play a very vital role in the future of cancer therapy as this receptor functions not as a single-target agent; conversely, it is involved in regulating multiple signaling pathways, which would ultimately translate in a complex cascade of events, affecting the growth and proliferative capabilities of cancer cells. This would represent a new therapeutic strategy, which might be able to overcome cancer resistance since multiple pathways are involved simultaneously. The advantage is that the modulation of this receptor might selectively challenge cancer tissues, since A₃ARs are known to be highly expressed in tumour cells as compared to normal cells. This would enable less undesired side effects (associated with conventional chemotherapy) and pave the way towards promising anticancer treatment.

4. A$_3$ ADENOSINE RECEPTOR AGONISTS

Adenosine (**1**), the endogenous ligand of adenosine receptors (ARs), binds to the hA$_3$AR subtype with a K$_i$ value of 290 nM [273]. To date, several A$_3$AR agonists, more potent and selective than adenosine, have been reported (Figure 7, Table 3). Most of these compounds derive from structural modifications of adenosine, although non-nucleoside derivatives have also been reported.

In order to obtain A$_3$AR agonists, adenosine can be modified at the adenine nucleus and/or at the ribose moiety. In particular, the adenine scaffold has been substituted at the N6 and C2 positions; usually, substitutions at the 5' position are the most common modifications on the ribose ring. Nevertheless, modifications of the pentose ring of ribose have also been reported, such as the substitution of the oxygen atom with a sulphur atom, or the replacement of the flexible ribose with a conformationally constrained bicycle [3.1.0] hexane ring (methanocarba).

After A$_3$AR was discovered and cloned in the '90s [4, 5], researchers investigated the unexplored structure-activity-relationship (SAR) profile for binding at A$_3$ARs. In a preliminary attempt to achieve selectivity at the A$_3$AR, van Galen et al. explored a wide range of adenosine derivatives for binding at the A$_3$AR. Concerning N6-aryl(alkyl)-substituted compounds, the authors found that N6-benzyladenosine was more potent (affinity at the (rat) A$_3$AR, rA$_3$AR, K$_i$ = 120 nM) than N6-phenyladenosine (rA$_3$ K$_i$ = 802 nM) or N6-phenethyladenosine (rA$_3$ K$_i$=240 nM) and displayed similar affinity at the rA$_1$ and rA$_2$ ARs, whereas the N6-phenyladenosine or N6-phenethyladenosine showed low nanomolar affinity at the rA$_1$AR [274]. NECA, (5'-N-ethylcarboxamide adenosine, (**2**) is a nonselective adenosine receptor agonist which displays good affinity also at the A$_3$AR (rA$_3$ K$_i$ = 113 nM). A$_3$AR affinity of NECA (**2**) is greater than the affinity of the natural ligand adenosine (**1**, hA$_3$ K$_i$ = 290 nM), thus indicating that the introduction of a N-ethylcarboxamide group at the 5' position enhances affinity at the A$_3$AR. Combination of the N6-benzyl moiety with the 5'-N-ethylcarboxamide group led to a potent and quite selective A$_3$AR agonist, N6-benzylNECA (rA$_3$ K$_i$ = 6.8 nM; hA$_3$ K$_i$ = 10.4 nM; rA$_1$/rA$_3$=13; rA$_{2A}$/rA$_3$ = 14) [274, 275]. Further exploration both on the benzyl group and on the uronamide moiety led to IB-MECA (**3**), which displays more potency (rA$_3$ K$_i$=1.1 nM; hA$_3$ K$_i$=1 nM) and selectivity (A$_1$/A$_3$ = r49, h51; A$_{2A}$/A$_3$=r51, h2, 900) than N6-benzylNECA [276]. Moreover, the effects of 2-substitution in combination with modifications at the N6 and 5' positions were explored. 2-Chloro-N6-(3-iodobenzyl)adenosine showed a K$_i$ value of 1.4 nM at rA$_3$AR and moderate selectivity for the other rat adenosine receptor subtypes, whereas 2-chloro-N6-(3-iodobenzyl)adenosine-5'-N-methyluronamide, Cl-IB-MECA (**4**), displayed a K$_i$ value of 0.33 nM at rA$_3$AR (hA$_3$ K$_i$=1.4 nM), and high selectivity against A$_1$ and A$_{2A}$ ARs (A$_1$/A$_3$=r2485, h159; A$_{2A}$/A$_3$=r1424, h3,829) [277]. IB-MECA (**3**) and Cl-IB-MECA (**4**) were also named CF100 and CF101 and they have been intensively used in preclinical and clinical studies for the treatment of various disorders and are the most representative A$_3$AR agonists [181, 215].

N6-Substitution Only

Gao et al. have carried out an intensive investigation at the N6 position of the unmodified-adenosine nucleus. Affinity at both human and rat A_3ARs, and efficacy at the hA_3AR were explored. Alkyl, cycloalkyl, aryl (or arylalkyl) and heteroaryl (or heteroarylalkyl) moieties were introduced at the N6 position [275]. In particular, small N6-alkyl groups gave selectivity for hA_3ARs *versus* rA_3ARs, whereas large or branched chains were associated with decreased hA_3AR efficacy. N6-arylmethyl groups generally displayed potency at the A_3AR, as well at the A_1AR. Further exploration on arylethyl analogues revealed a strong steric control at the N6 position, which influenced efficacy, affinity and selectivity of the derivatives. The N6-[(1S,2R)-2-phenyl-1-cyclopropyl]adenosine (**5**) showed a K_i value of 9.63 nM toward the hA_3AR and a 1100-fold selectivity against the rA_3AR (Figure 7, Table 3). Unfortunately, all these compounds still retain high affinity also at the A_1AR [275]. Starting from the IB-MECA (**3**) structure, Baraldi et al. explored substitutions at the N6 position with urea moieties (particularly N-phenylureas). Derivatives were all potent at the rA_3AR, but not selective, especially towards the rA_1AR [278].

C2 Substitution

Volpini et al. have investigated the C2 position by introducing alkynyl moieties [279, 280]. Initially, they introduced alkynyl groups at the C2 position of adenosine (**1**) and NECA (**2**). Generally, adenosine derivatives showed higher activity at the A_1AR and lower activity at the A_3 and A_{2A} ARs than NECA derivatives. PENECA (2-phenylethynyl-adenosine-5'-N-ethyluronamide, **6**) is the C2-phenylethynyl derivative of NECA, although its affinity at the hA_3AR is the same of NECA (hA_3 K_i=6.2 nM), it showed a remarkable increased selectivity towards A_1 and A_{2A} ARs [279]. Alkylation of the amino group at the 6 position of adenosine with a little methyl group, increased affinity at the A_3AR and had a detrimental effect on affinities at the other ARs, thus enhancing selectivity toward A_3AR. In particular, compound **7**, HEMADO (2-hexyn-1-yl-N6-methyladenosine), which bears a hexynyl moiety at the C2 position, showed a K_i value of 1.1 nM at the hA_3AR and a selectivity of about 300 and 1'100 times against A_1 and A_{2A} ARs, respectively [280]. HEMADO (**7**) was chosen for the development of a radioligand selective for the A_3AR. Its tritiated form, [^{3}H]HEMADO, was obtained by substitution of the iodine of 2-(hexyn-1-yl)-6-iodo-purine-9-riboside with tritiated methylamine. [^{3}H]HEMADO displays high affinity and selectivity at the A_3AR and very low nonspecific binding, therefore it is a useful tool for specific screening for hA_3AR agonists and antagonists in improved radioligand binding assays [281].

Successively, the same group and others [282, 283, 284] have developed series in which different kinds of substitutions were introduced on the ethynyl group at C2 position with N-methyl or N-ethyl uronamides at the 5' position and with methyl, ethyl or methoxy moieties at the N6 position. Compounds **8** and **9** are the most interesting compounds in terms of both affinity and selectivity at the hA_3AR (Figure 7).

Besides (ar)alkynyl moieties, other substitutions were also explored at the C2 position of the adenine scaffold. Ohno et al. developed a series of N6-(aryl)alkyladenosine derivatives substituted with little groups at the C2 position such as cyano, amino, aminomethyl, carboxyl, carboxamido or trifluoromethyl groups [285]. Except for the cyano group, all the other groups inserted at the C2 position were detrimental for affinity at the A$_3$AR compared to the unsubstituted compounds. On the other hand, the cyano group at the C2 position gave different effects on the base of N6-substituent. C2-cyano moiety is beneficial when a little alkyl group is introduced at the N6 position (compound **10**), whereas it decreases affinity at the hA$_3$AR in derivatives bearing a large group at the N6 position, such as the 3-iodobenzyl or the *trans*-2-phenyl-1-cyclopropyl moieties.

Finally, five ring heterocycles such as triazoles and pyrazoles were introduced at the C2 position to explore their effect on binding at the A$_3$AR [282, 286]. C2-Pyrazol-1-yl derivatives were extensively explored by Zablocky et al. in CV Therapeutics. On the basis of previous results obtained by Volpini et al. on the 2-alkynyl adenosine analogues [280], the authors decided to investigate the effect of introducing substituents at the N6-position of 2-pyrazolyl adenosine analogues, which were potent and selective A$_{2A}$AR agonists, with the idea of identifying new high affinity and selective A$_3$AR agonists. Pyrazole ring was substituted with various heteroaryl groups. Potent and selective A$_3$AR agonists were obtained when a methyl group was present at the N6 position (as demonstrated by Volpini et al.) and one of the best compounds of the series is derivative **11** (hA$_3$ K$_i$ = 2 nM), which bears a 4-(pyridin-2-yl)-pyrazol-1-yl group at the C2 position [286].

Ribose Modification

The first modification of the ribose ring that has been found to confer high affinity at the hA$_3$AR is the introduction of a *N*-alkyluronamide moiety at the 5' position, such as in IB-MECA (**3**) and Cl-IB-MECA (**4**) [276, 277, 287]. Furthermore, the 5'-uronamide moiety may be constricted in an isoxazole ring without detrimental effects on affinity at the A$_3$AR, such as for compound **12** [288]. 2'-Deoxy and 3'-deoxy adenosine displayed low affinity at the A$_3$AR, demonstrating that the 2'-OH and the 3'-OH are essential for high affinity [274]. In the attempt to search for selective hA$_3$AR agonists useful for the prevention of perioperative myocardial ischemia, Pfizer discovered CP-608039 (**13**). CP-608039 (**13**) contains an amino group instead of a hydroxy group at the 3' position of ribose ring; this modification confers high selectivity for the hA$_3$AR against the hA$_1$AR (hA$_1$/hA$_3$=1,260) [289].

In 2003, Jeong et al. reported a series of 4'-thioadenosine derivatives [290]. The substitution of the adenosine nucleus in Cl-IB-MECA (**4**) with a 4'-thioadenosine gave derivative LJ-529 (LJ568, **14**), which acts as a highly potent and selective A$_3$AR full agonist with a subnanomolar affinity (hA$_3$ K$_i$ = 0.38 nM). Further explorations on N6-substituted-4'-thioadenosines led to the achievement of a SAR profile of these derivatives at the hA$_3$AR: N6-methyl moiety is beneficial both for affinity and selectivity; 4'-thioadenosine derivatives show higher affinity than the corresponding 4'-oxoadenosine derivatives at the hA$_3$AR; 5'-uronamide moiety enhances affinity at the hA$_3$AR. One of the most potent and selective 4'-thioadenosine derivatives is LJ-530 (**15**) which shows the same affinity at the hA$_3$AR as LJ-529 (hA$_3$ K$_i$ = 0.28 nM) but a higher selectivity versus the other AR subtypes (hA$_1$/hA$_3$=4,750; hA$_{2A}$/hA$_3$>35,714) [290, 291, 292, 293].

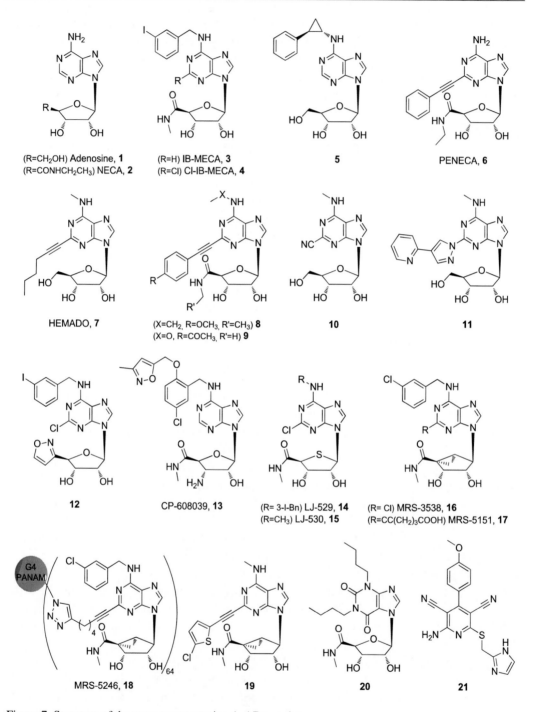

Figure 7. Structure of the most representative A_3AR agonists.

Table 3. Binding affinities of the most representative A₃AR agonists at the A₁, A₂A, A₂B and A₃ ARs

Compound	A₁ AR K_i (nM) or % of displ.[a]	A₂A AR K_i (nM) or % of displ.[a]	A₂B AR EC_{50} (nM) or % of act.[b]	A₃ AR K_i (nM)[c]	A₁/A₃	A₂A/A₃
1, Adenosine [273]	310^d	730^d	23,500	290^d	~1	2.4
2, NECA [274, 279]	13.6 (r) 6.3	20.1 (r) 10.3	2,360	6.2 (r) 113	2.2 (r) 0.1	3.2 (r) 0.1
3, IB-MECA [277, 279]	3.73 (r) 54	2,520 (r) 56	11,000	1.2 (r) 1.1	3 (r) 49	2,100 (r) 51
4, Cl-IB-MECA [277, 279]	115 (r) 820	2,100 (r) 470	> 100,000	11.1 (r) 0.33	10 (r) 2,485	187 (r) 1,424
5 [275]	(r) 11.8	(r) 560	n.d.	0.63 (r) 694	(r) 0.02	(r) 0.81
6, PENECA [279]	560	620	n.d.	6.2	90	100
7, HEMADO [280]	327	1,230	n.d.	1.1	297	1118
8 [283]	558	4,963	n.d.	0.75	746	6,635
9 [284]	53,800	10,400	n.d.	2.5	3,600	16,400
10 [285]	69.8	23% (10 µM)	n.d.	3.4	20.5	> 2,941
11 [286]	3,800	> 5,000	n.d.	2	1,900	> 2,000
12 [288]	(r) 1,900	(r) 1,900	n.d.	7.8	-	-
13, CP-608039 [289]	7,300	n.d.	n.d.	5.8	1,260	-
14, LJ-529 [290]	193^l (r) 140	223 (r) 348	n.d.	0.38	508	587
15, LJ-530 [290]	1,330 (r) 198	20% (10 µM) (r) 6,340	n.d.	0.28	4,750	> 35,714
16, MRS-3558 [297, 298]	260 (m) 15.3	2,300 (m) 10,400	38% (10 µM)	0.29 (m) 1.49 (r) 1.0	897 (m) 10.3	7,931 (m) 6,980
17, MRS-5151 [298]	14,900 (m) 10,500	43% (10 µM) (m) 8% (100 µM)	n.d.	2.38 (m) 24.4	6,260 (m) 430	> 4,202
18, MRS-5246 [304, 305]	22.6 (m) 14.35	32.2	n.d.	0.14 (m) 0.04	161 (m) 359	230
19 [302]	6% (10 µM) (m) 30% (10 µM)	24% (10 µM) (m) 7% (10 µM)	n.d.	0.7 (m) 36.1	> 14,286 (m) 277	> 14,286 (m) 277
20 [308]	(r) 37,300	(r) 19% (100 µM)	n.d.	(r) 229	(r) 163	(r) > 437)
21 [306]	7.0	214	9	24	0.3	8.9

^{a} Displacement of specific radioligand binding, unless noted, in human ARs, expressed as K_i values or % of displacement. A percent value indicates the percent displacement of radioligand at the concentration given in parentheses. (m): mouse; (r): rat. ^{b}cAMP assay in CHO cells expressing human A₂B adenosine receptors. A percent value indicates the percent stimulation of cAMP levels at the concentration given in parentheses. ^{c}Displacement of specific radioligand binding, unless noted, in human ARs, expressed as K_i values. (m): mouse; (r): rat. ^{d}EC₅₀ values.

Among the ribose modifications, Jacobson and co-workers reported a series of congeners of potent A_3AR nucleoside agonists containing a bicyclo[3.1.0]hexane ring [294, 295, 296, 297, 298, 299, 300, 301, 302]. This ring resembles to the north conformation of ribose that was found to be preferred conformation for binding to the ARs [294]. 5'-Uronamide derivatives are selective A_3AR agonists, on the contrary, 4'-truncated derivatives display an antagonistic activity [303]. MRS-3558 (CF502, **16**) is an example of potent A_3AR agonist of this series in both human (hA_3 K_i=0.29 nM) and rat (rA_3 K_i=1 nM) receptors. The substitution of the chlorine at the C2 position of MRS-3558 (**16**) with a hex-5-ynoic acid increases the selectivity versus both A_1 and A_{2A} ARs (MRS-5151, **17**) (hA_1/hA_3=6,260; hA_{2A}/hA_3>4,202) [298, [297]. The presence of a carboxylic group in MRS-5151 (**17**) and its analogues, has been used to the conjugation with alkyldiamines, which serve as spacers for the final introduction of fluorescent dyes or biotin [300]. Instead, C2-dialkynyl or N6-propargyl derivatives were coupled by click reaction with azido derivatives of fourth-generation multivalent poly(amidoamine) (PAMAM) dendrimers, to form [1, 2, 3] triazolyl linkers. The conjugation between ligands and dendrimers could prevent their *in vivo* premature degradation or even enhance tissue selectivity, furthermore it could greatly improve potency or effectiveness of the ligands. MRS-5246 (**18**) proved to be effective in increasing functional recovery of isolated mouse hearts after 20 minutes of ischemia followed by 45 minutes of reperfusion [304, 305]. Similarly to those reported by Volpini et al., the introduction of rigid extended C2-arylalkynyl groups in (N)-methanocarba adenosine derivatives is well tolerated at the hA_3AR. In addition, small groups at the N6 position (i.e., methyl) give derivatives which are typically more potent at the hA_3AR than at the rA_3AR. The highly potent A_3AR agonist, compound **19**, shows high efficacy in reversing chronic neuropathic pain in mouse, with a long *in vivo* duration [302].

Finally, few examples of non-adenosine based A_3AR agonists have been reported. In particular, Kim et al. [277, 287] reported a series of 1,3-dialkylxanthine-7-riboside derivatives in which the xanthinic scaffold is introduced in place of the adenine ring of adenosine nucleoside. Only a few compounds displayed affinity at the rA_3AR in the high nanomolar range, such as compound **20** (rA_3 K_i=229 nM). An example of non-nucleosidic A_3AR agonist is the pyridine derivative, compound **21**, discovered by Beukers et al. [306]. Compound **21**, as all the other derivatives reported in this work, is a non-selective agonist for the ARs, but it could represent the starting point for the development of non-nucleoside selective A_3AR agonists. In addition, compound **21** displays only 39% of efficacy in the inhibition of cAMP production as compared to the reference agonist Cl-IB-MECA, thus it behaves as a partial agonist.

5. A_3 ADENOSINE RECEPTOR ANTAGONISTS

The natural adenosine receptor antagonists are the xanthines caffeine (**22**) and theophylline (**23**), which are neither potent nor selective for any adenosine receptor subtype, [ref] but have represented the starting point to develop more potent and selective adenosine receptor antagonists (Figure 8, Table 4). As for the other ARs, both xanthine-based and non-xanthine-based derivatives have been designed as A_3AR antagonists. Several non-xanthine-based A_3AR antagonists have been reported which can be classified, on the base of the number of cycles that form the central scaffold of the derivative, in: tricyclic derivatives; bicyclic derivatives and monocyclic derivatives.

Xanthine-Based Derivatives

Generally, xanthine derivatives do not display high affinity towards the human A_3AR. The introduction of a phenyl ring at the 8 position, along with a large substituent at the 3 position, of the xanthine scaffold enhances affinity at the hA_3AR, such as for I-ABOPX (24). I-ABOPX (24) possesses a K_i value of 15 nM at the hA_3AR, although it lacks of selectivity versus the other AR subtypes [37, 277, 287, 307, 308, 309].

Table 4. Binding affinities of the xanthine-based A_3AR antagonists at the A_1, A_{2A}, A_{2B} and A_3 ARs

Compound	A_1 AR K_i (nM) or % of displ.[a]	A_{2A} AR K_i (nM) or % of displ.[a]	A_{2B} AR IC_{50} (nM)[b]	A_3 AR K_i (nM)[c]	A_1/A_3	A_{2A}/A_3
22, Caffeine [ref]	10,700	9,560	10,400[d]	13,300	0.80	0.72
23, Theophylline [ref]	6,920	6,700	9,070[d]	22,300	0.31	0.30
24, I-ABOPX [277, 309]	70 (r) 37	95 (r) 700	40[d]	15 (r) 1170 (s) 2	4.6 (r) 0.03	6.3 (r) 0.60
25 [311]	24% (1 μM)	0% (1 μM)	> 1,000[d]	2.24	> 446	> 446
26 [312]	> 1,000	> 1,000	> 1,000	3.5	> 290	> 290
27 [312]	> 1,000	> 1,000	> 1,000	0.8	> 1,250	> 1,250
28, PSB-11 [314, 315]	1,640 (r) 440	1,280 (r) 2,100	(m) 2,100[e]	2.3	713	556
29, PSB-10 [315]	1,700 (r) 805	2,700 (r) 6,040	n.d.	0.43	3,953	6,279
30, KF-26777 [316]	1,800	470	620[d]	0.20	9,000	2,350
32 [318]	2,525	> 5,000	> 5,000	1.46	1,729	> 3425

[a] Displacement of specific radioligand binding, unless noted, in human ARs, expressed as K_i values or % of displacement. A percent value indicates the percent displacement of radioligand at the concentration given in parentheses. (m): mouse; (r): rat. [b]Potency of examined compounds to inhibit stimulation of cAMP levels (cAMP assay) in CHO cells expressing $hA_{2B}ARs$, expressed as IC_{50}. [c]Displacement of specific radioligand binding, unless noted, in human ARs, expressed as K_i values. (m): mouse; (r): rat. [d]Displacement of [^{125}I]-ABOPX (22-25) or [^{3}H]DPCPX (30) radioligand binding in HEK-293 cell membrane expressing human $A_{2B}ARs$, expressed as K_i values [e]cAMP assay in NIH 3T3 fibroblast cell membranes. Binding to $A_{2B}AR$ is expressed with K_B value calculated from IC_{50} value.

The condensation of the xanthine ring system with a third ring between positions 7 and 8, such as a pyridine (e.g., compound 25) [310, 311], pyrrole (e.g., compound 26) or an imidazole (e.g., compound 27) [312, 313], led to highly potent hA_3AR antagonists with enhanced selectivity towards ARs. Instead, the condensation of an imidazole ring at the 1 and the 6 positions of the xanthine nucleus is a strategy previously used to enhance solubility of A_1AR antagonists. In fact, the basic nitrogen atom of imidazole ring can be protonated under physiological conditions, conferring a better water-solubility of these imadazolepurines compared to xanthine derivatives. The same strategy applied to A_3AR antagonists led to the development of the imidazolepurin-5-one derivatives, PSB-11 (**28**), PSB-10 (**29**) and KF-26777 (**30**) [314, 315, 316]. The introduction of an alkyl moiety at the 6 position of the imidazolepurin-5-one derivatives gives chiral compounds and a slight level of enantioselectivity was observed concerning affinity at the rA_1 and hA_3 ARs.

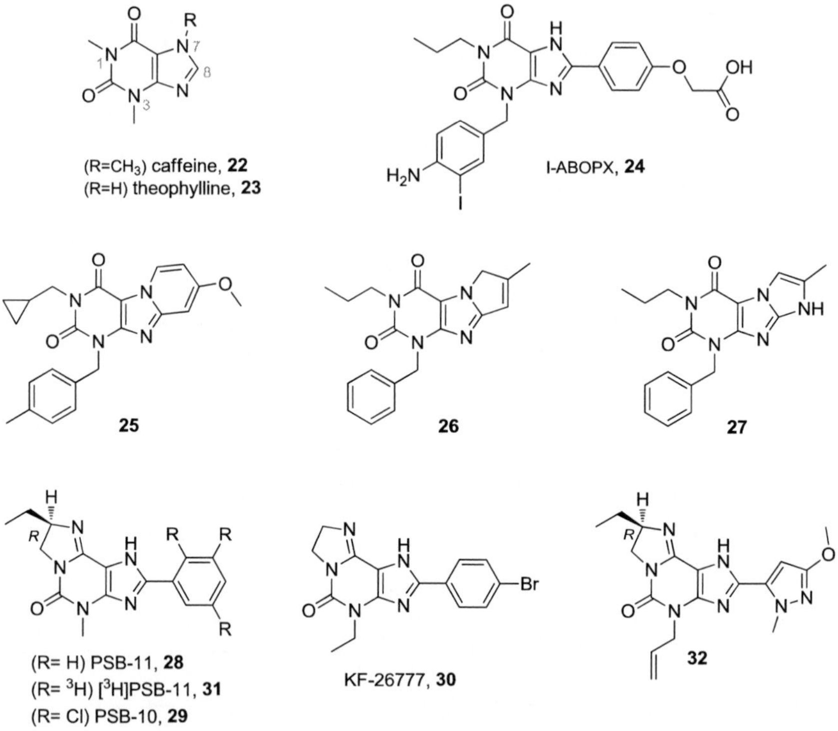

Figure 8. Structure of xanthine-based A_3AR antagonists.

In particular, (R)-enantiomers show higher affinity at the hA_3AR and less affinity at the rA_1AR than (S)-enantiomers. Therefore, (R)-enantiomers displayed enhanced affinity but especially they displayed enhanced selectivity at the A_3AR [314, 315]. PSB-11 (**28**) was developed also in its tritiated form as antagonist radioligand for the hA_3AR. [^{3}H]PSB-11 (**31**) was prepared by catalytic hydrogenation of the trichlorophenyl precursor PSB-10 (**29**) using tritium gas [317]. KF-26777 (**30**) is now under preclinical investigation as anti-asthmatic agent. The phenyl moiety at the 2 position of the imidazolepurin-5-one can also be substituted with isoxazolyl or pyrazolyl rings, which induce excellent affinity and selectivity toward hA_3AR subtype (**32**) [318].

Tricyclic Derivatives

CGS-15943 (**33**) is a [1, 2, 4]triazolo[1,5-c]quinazoline derivative discovered in 1988 as an adenosine receptor antagonist (Figure 9) [319]. CGS-15943 (**33**) shows K_i affinity values in the nanomolar range at the rA$_1$, rA$_{2A}$ and hA$_3$ ARs, whereas it is inactive at the rA$_3$AR. Therefore, the [1, 2, 4] triazolo[1,5-c]quinazoline scaffold was used as template for the development of potent and selective hA$_3$AR antagonists, such as MRS-1220 (**34**). In fact, acylation of the free amino group at the N5 position of CGS-15943 with benzoyl or phenyacetyl moieties led to an improvement of affinity and selectivity at the hA$_3$AR (e.g., MRS-1220, **34** hA$_3$ K$_i$ = 0.65 nM; rA$_1$/hA$_3$ = 81.1; rA$_{2A}$/hA$_3$ > 15.8) [320]. The substitution of the 2-furyl ring with a *para*-methoxyphenyl group, and the introduction of a butyl moiety in place of the 5-amino group of CGS-15943, led to compound **35**, which displays a K$_i$ of 160 nM at the hA$_3$AR and selectivity more than 62-fold against A$_1$ and A$_{2A}$ ARs [321]. Kozma et al. [322] have developed a fluorescent A$_3$AR antagonists, MRS-5449 (**36**), prepared using a click reaction between a [1, 2, 4]triazolo[1,5-c]quinazoline derivative and a derivative of the fluorescent dye Alexa Fluor 488. MRS-5449 (**36**) shows high affinity at the hA$_3$AR (K$_i$ = 6.4 nM) and has been used successfully in quantifying the hA$_3$AR, studying receptor kinetic properties, and ligand screening in intact cells using flow cytometry.

In 1993, Gatta et al. tried to modify the [1, 2, 4]triazolo[1,5-c]quinazoline core of CGS-15943 in order to improve selectivity towards the A$_{2A}$AR. Authors have synthesized analogues in which the phenyl group was replaced by a heterocyclic ring such as pyrazole, leading to the pyrazolo[4,3-e] [1, 2, 4]triazolo[1,5-c]pyrimidine derivatives. Because small variations in the [1, 2, 4]triazolo[1,5-c]quinazoline scaffold of CGS-15943 improve affinity at the A$_3$AR, the same strategy was applied on the pyrazolo[4,3-e] [1, 2, 4]triazolo[1,5-c]pyrimidine nucleus. In fact, aryl-, arylalkyl- amides or arylureas at the 5 position, with a little alkyl group at the N8 position (i.e., methyl) and the 2-furyl ring at the 2 position gave potent and selective hA$_3$AR antagonists [323, 324, 325, 326, 327]. The most potent pyrazolo[4,3-e][1, 2, 4]triazolo[1,5-c]pyrimidine derivative is compound **37** (hA$_3$ K$_i$ = 0.01 nM), which shows also a good water-solubility for the presence of a pyridinium ring [326]. Another representative compound of this class of derivatives is MRE-3008-F20 (**38**), a highly selective hA$_3$AR antagonist that can be obtained also in its tritiated form, [^{3}H]MRE-3008-F20 (**39**), and it is currently used for pharmacological studies involving hA$_3$AR [323, 328]. Recently, new discoveries on the SAR of the pyrazolo[4,3-e][1,2,4]triazolo[1,5-c]pyrimidine at the hA$_3$AR have been reported. Cheong et al. have found that the 2-furyl ring at the 2 position can be replaced by a phenyl ring leading to a substantial improvement of selectivity against the other AR subtypes (e.g., compound **40**, hA$_3$ K$_i$ = 0.24 nM; hA$_1$/hA$_3$ > 124,000; hA$_{2A}$/hA$_3$ > 415,000) [329]. Whereas, Federico et al. have reported that pyrazolo[4,3-e][1,2,4]triazolo[1,5-c]pyrimidine bearing different (ar)alkylamino moieties instead of amidic or ureidic groups at the 5 position are still able to bind the hA$_3$AR with high affinity (hA$_3$ K$_i$ = 0.3 nM) and also high selectivity (hA$_1$/hA$_3$ > 1,127; hA$_{2A}$/hA$_3$ > 184), such as compound **41** (Figure 9, Table 5) [330].

The [1, 2, 4]triazolo[5,1-i]purine scaffold is structurally related to the pyrazolo[4,3-e][1, 2 ,4]triazolo[1,5-c]pyrimidine nucleus, in which the triazole ring is directly incorporated on the purine ring, between positions 1 and 6 [321]. OT-7999 (**42**) is the most representative compound of the series and it is very potent and selective for the hA$_3$AR subtype. It resembles to the triazoloquinazoline derivative **35**, in fact, it bears a phenyl ring at the 8 position with a butyl moiety at the 5 position. OT-7999 (**42**) significantly reduced intraocular pressure compared with the control eye, thus indicating its potential application in the treatment of glaucoma [331].

In the last years, several other tricyclic scaffolds structurally related to CGS-15943 (**33**) were reported as templates for the design of new potent and selective hA_3 AR: [1, 2, 4]triazolo[4,3-*a*]quinoxalines (e.g., compounds **43-45**, Figure 9, Table 5) [332, 333, 334, 335, 336, 337], [1,2,4]triazolo[1,5-*a*]quinoxalines (e.g., compound **46**) [338, 339], pyrazolo[3,4-*c*]quinolines (e.g., compounds **47-48**) [332, 340], pyrazolo[4,3-*c*]quinolines (e.g., compound **49**) [341], pyrido[2,3-*e*][1,2,4]triazolo[4,3-*a*]pyrazin-1-one (e.g., compound **50**) [342] and [1,2,3]triazolo[1,2-*a*][1,2,4]benzotriazin-1-one (e.g., compound **51**) [343] are the most representative (Figure 10, Table 5). All these class of compounds display few conservative features that confer them affinity and selectivity toward the hA_3AR subtypes. The introduction of a carbonyl group at the 4 position (5 position in triazolobenzotriazinone series), either by acylation of the 4-amino group with alkanoyl, aryloyl or arylalkanoyl moieties, or by replacement of the amino group with an oxo group, appeared essential for hA_3AR affinity and selectivity.

Table 5. Binding affinities of the tricyclic A_3AR antagonists at the A_1, A_{2A}, A_{2B} and A_3 ARs

Compound	A_1 AR K_i (nM) or % of displ.[a]	A_{2A} AR K_i (nM) or % of displ.[a]	A_{2B} AR IC_{50} (nM) or % of inhib.[b]	A_3 AR K_i (nM)[c]	A_1/A_3	A_{2A}/A_3
33, CGS15943 [320, 1]	3.5 (r) 21	1.2 (r) 3.3	1,200	13.8	0.25	0.09
34, MRS-1220 [320]	(r) 52.7	(r) 10.3	71% (50 µM)	0.65	-	-
35 [321]	n.d.	> 10,000[d]	n.d.	160[d]	-	62.5
36, MRS-5449 [322]	87.0	73.0	n.d.	6.4	13.6	11.4
37 [326]	350	100	250[e]	0.01	35,000	10,000
38, MRE3008-F20 [323, 325]	1,197 (r) > 10,000	141 (r) 1,993	2,056[e]	0.8 (r) 37% (10 mM)	1,496	175
40 [329]	> 30,000	> 100,000	> 10,000[f]	0.24	> 124,000	> 415,000
41 [330]	338	55.2	5,290[f]	0.3	1,127	184
42, OT-7999 [331]	> 10,000[d]	> 10,000[d]	> 10,000[e]	0.61[d]	> 16,393	> 16,393
43 [334]	32% (10 µM) (b) 19% (20 µM)	(b) 21% (20 µM)	n.d.	0. 6	> 16,667	-
44 [335]	11% (10 µM) (b) 260	2% (10 µM) (b) 0% (10 µM)	n.d.	0.8	> 12,500	> 12,500
45 [337]	27,542[g]	n.d.	> 1,000[g]	43.6[g]	632	-
46 [338]	(b) 127	(b) 0% (20 µM)	n.d.	0.5	-	-
47 [340]	29.0 (b) 3,900	44% (10 µM) (b) 32% (20 µM)	n.d.	3.2	9.1	> 3,125
48 [340]	25% (10 µM)	7% (10 µM)	n.d.	17.2	> 581	> 581
49 [341]	> 1,000	> 1,000	> 1,000	9.0	> 111	> 111

Table 5. (Continued)

Compound	A$_1$ AR K$_i$ (nM) or % of displ.[a]	A$_{2A}$ AR K$_i$ (nM) or % of displ.[a]	A$_{2B}$ AR IC$_{50}$ (nM) or % of inhib.[b]	A$_3$ AR K$_i$ (nM)[c]	A$_1$/A$_3$	A$_{2A}$/A$_3$
50 [342]	38% (10 μM) (b) 355	27% (10 μM) (b) 7% (20 μM)	n.d.	4.54	> 2,202	> 2,202
51 [343]	2,700	> 10,000	> 1,000	1.6	1,687	> 6,250

[a] Displacement of specific radioligand binding, unless noted, in human ARs, expressed as K$_i$ values or % of displacement. A percent value indicates the percent displacement of radioligand at the concentration given in parentheses. (b): bovine; (r): rat. [b]Potency of examined compounds to inhibit stimulation of cAMP levels (cAMP assay) in CHO cells expressing hA$_{2B}$ARs, expressed as IC$_{50}$. A percent value indicates the percent inhibition of stimulated cAMP levels at the concentration given in parentheses. [c]Displacement of specific radioligand binding, unless noted, in human ARs, expressed as K$_i$ values. (r): rat.[d]IC$_{50}$ values. [e]Displacement of specific [^{3}H]DPCPX binding at hA$_{2B}$ receptors expressed in HEK-293, in membranes. [f]K$_i$ values of the inhibition of NECA-stimulated adenylyl cyclase activity in CHO cells. [g]Functional assays, binding affinities are expressed as K$_D$, antagonist equilibrium dissociation constant.

These findings highlight the importance for the ligand-A$_3$AR interaction of both a strong acidic NH proton donor and a C = O proton acceptor near the position 4 (5 for compound **51**) of the above mentioned tricyclic scaffolds, which are able to engage hydrogen-bonding interactions with specific residues inside the A$_3$AR binding cleft. Another common feature among these class of compounds is the presence of a phenyl ring at the 2 position; substitutions on the phenyl ring are able to modulate both affinity and selectivity at the hA$_3$AR [344, 333, 334, 335, 336].

Vernall et al. developed a highly potent and selective fluorescent antagonists of the hA$_3$AR based on the [1, 2, 4]triazolo[4,3-*a*]quinoxalin-1-one scaffold, using BODIPY-X-630/650 as fluorescent probe (e.g., compound **45**, hA$_3$ K$_D$ = 43.6 nM). Compound **45** demonstrated to be an effective biological probe for optical-based experiments [337]. Recently, some potent [1,2,4]triazolo[4,3-*a*]quinoxalin-1-one derivatives, such as compound **44**, were radiolabeled with carbon-11 for PET (positron emission tomography) imaging of A$_3$ ARs (Figure 9, Table 5) [345].

Bicyclic Derivatives

The first bicyclic scaffold reported as a template for the design of A$_3$AR antagonists was the flavonoid nucleus. The discovery that flavonoid derivatives have slight affinity towards the A$_3$AR was due to a screening of phytochemicals libraries [346].

Subsequently, a structural optimization on the flavone nucleus led to MRS-1067 (**52**), which displays a K$_i$ value of 561 nM at the hA$_3$AR and a good selectivity profile against the other AR subtypes (rA$_1$/hA$_3$ > 178; rA$_{2A}$/hA$_3$ > 178). As for the other A$_3$AR antagonists thus far reported, MRS-1067 (**52**) displays selectivity for the human versus the rat A$_3$AR, in fact, functional assay at the rA$_3$AR reveals a K$_i$ value of 5.5 μM (Figure 11, Table 6) [347, 348].

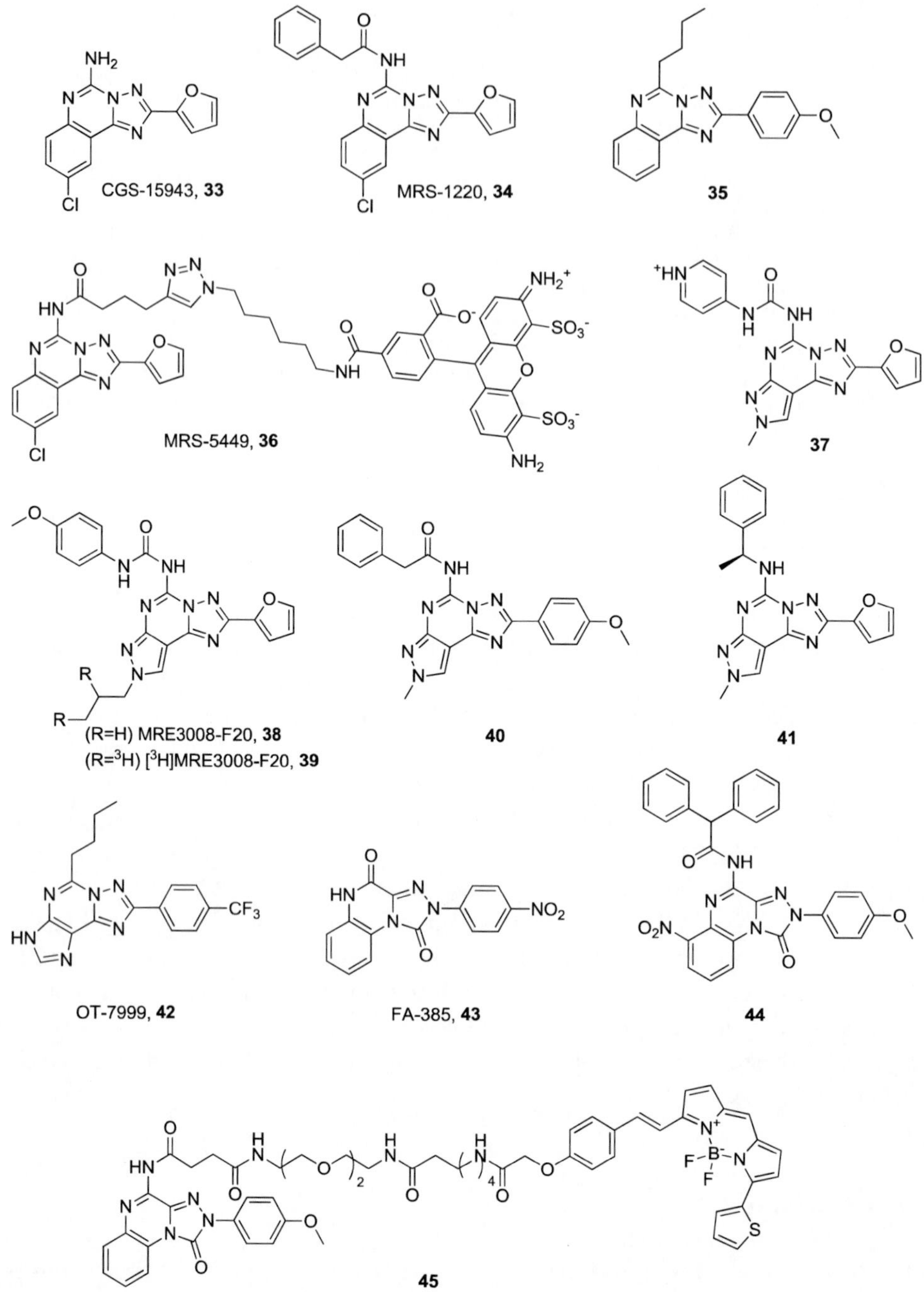

Figure 9. Structure of tricyclic A₃AR antagonists. Compounds **33-45.**

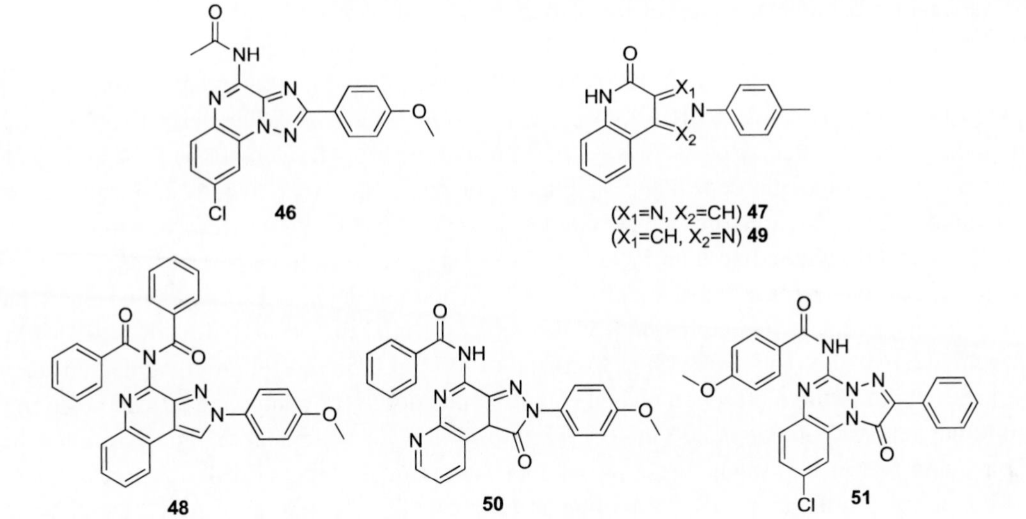

Figure 10. Structure of tricyclic A$_3$ AR antagonists. Compounds **46-51.**

A CoMFA (Comparative Molecular Field Analysis) analysis on this class of derivatives at the ARs addressed the steric and/or electrostatic requirements for ligand binding: a phenyl ring at the 2 position is important for interaction with all the AR subtypes, whereas substituents at the 2' and 6 positions are well tolerated at the A$_3$AR, leading to an enhancement of selectivity at this AR subtype [349]. Recently, Borges F. group have investigated the coumarin scaffold for affinity at the hA$_3$AR, but obtained derivatives do not display appreciable potency and selectivity for the target [350].

van Muijlwijk-Koezen et al. reported two classes of hA$_3$AR antagonists bearing isoquinoline and quinazoline nuclei, respectively [351, 352, 353]. VUF-8504 (**53**) and VUF-5574 (**54**) are the most representative compounds of these two series. They are very similar in their structure; in fact, both of them bear a pyridyl moiety at the 3 (2-pyridyl) and 2 (3-pyridyl) positions of the isoquinoline and quinazoline core, respectively. At the 1 position, VUF-8504 (**53**) presents a 4-methoxybenzamido group, whereas, at the corresponding position on the VUF-5574 (**54**) (position 4 of quinazoline) a 2-methoxyphenylureido moiety is present. At a later stage, VUF-8504 (**53**) was found to exert also as a positive allosteric modulator at the hA$_3$AR [354]. Nevertheless, SAR analysis has revealed the allosteric effects were separable from competitive antagonism, thus promoting the development of allosteric modulators without antagonistic activity (Figure 11, Table 6).

Moro and co. applied the concept of molecular simplification on the [1, 2, 4]triazolo[4,3-*a*]quinoxaline scaffold [355]. Simplified quinazoline, quinoxaline and pyrimidine derivatives have been synthesized. Only the quinazoline derivatives display affinity in the nanomolar range at the hA$_3$AR, the most potent compound (compound **55**) exhibits a structure similarity to compounds reported by IJzerman and co. (**53**, **54**) [355]. Analogously, the same research groups developed the phtalazyn-1(2H)-one derivatives. Even in this case, a potent and selective hA$_3$AR has been discovered, compound **56**. Molecular docking studies on [1, 2, 4]triazolo[4,3-*a*]quinoxaline, quinazoline and phtalazyn-1(2H)-one derivatives confirmed a similar binding mode of these compounds as was expected from the simplification approach [356].

Pyrazolopyrimidines represent interesting simplified scaffolds of the more complex, but highly potent, tricyclic classes of hA$_3$AR antagonists. Colotta and co. investigated the pyrazolo[4,3-d]pyrimidine scaffold [357, 358], whereas Taliani et al. explored the pyrazolo[3,4-d]pyrimidine nucleus [359]. The pyrazolo[4,3-d]pyrimidine derivative **57** shows a binding affinity value, expressed as K$_i$, of 24 nM at the hA$_3$AR. Compound **57** significantly prevent the oxaliplatin-dependent apoptosis of rat astrocytes when co-incubated at micromolar concentration, thus suggesting a protective effect on astrocytes. Nevertheless, the complete inactivity of compound **57** at the rA$_3$AR suggests an A$_3$-independent mechanism of action [358]. Concerning the pyrazolo [3,4-d] pyrimidine derivatives, compound **58** is the most potent and selective compound of the series towards the hA$_3$AR (hA$_3$ K$_i$ = 0.18 nM; hA$_1$/hA$_3$=5761; hA$_{2A}$/hA$_3$=17,661). Compounds **57** and **58** are highly similar in their structure; both of them present a phenyl ring (i.e., position 5 for compound **57** and position 6 for compound **58**) and an amido moiety (i.e., position 7 for compound **57** and position 4 for compound **58**) in equivalent positions of their structure. Compound **58** was tested for its effect on the proliferation of U87MG human glioma cells. The reference A$_3$AR agonists IB-MECA (**3**) and Cl-IB-MECA (**4**) were able to stimulate U87MG cell proliferation. This effect is contrasted by compound **58**, however, it is unable to modulate U87MG cell proliferation alone [359].

Considering that several classes of A$_3$AR agonists and antagonists have a N-phenylcarbamoyl function, Biagi et al. decided to introduce this moiety at the 7 position of the [1, 2, 3]triazolo[4,5-d]pyrimidine nucleus. A structural optimization by little modifications at the 3, 5 and 7 positions led to the discovery of compound **59**, which displays affinity at the hA$_3$AR in the nanomolar range (K$_i$ = 6 nM) [360].

The purine ring obviously represents an interesting scaffold for search new potent AR antagonists. Volpini et al. have reported several 9-alkyladenine derivatives. Compounds selectivity relies on substitutions at the 2 and 8 positions [361, 362]. The 9-ethyl-9H-adenine derivative **60**, bearing a phenylethynyl moiety at the 8 position, is a quite selective hA$_3$AR antagonist (hA$_3$ K$_i$ = 86 nM; hA$_1$/hA$_3$ = 15; hA$_{2A}$/hA$_3$ = 7). In addition, compound **60** displays a comparable affinity also at the rat A$_3$ subtype, which made compound **60** a good pharmacological tool for studies on rats [362]. Perreira et al. synthesized different 2,6-disubstituted adenine derivatives and identified a highly selective hA$_3$AR antagonist, the 2-phenoxy-N6-cyclohexyladenine, MRS-3777 (**61**), which shows a binding affinity in the nanomolare range (K$_i$ = 47 nM) [363].

As clearly depicted in section 4 (4. A$_3$ Adenosine Receptor Agonists), adenosine derivatives are principally developed as adenosine receptor agonists. An advantage of adenosine derivatives is that generally bind indiscriminately different species of receptors. Some structural modifications on the ribose ring lead to an improvement of affinity at the hA$_3$AR and enhance stability in biological systems. Nevertheless, modifications of adenosine structure may affect the efficacy of the agonists at the hA$_3$AR and even antagonist can be obtained. Gao et al. have investigated the structural features that cause activation or inactivation of the hA$_3$AR [296]. The study shows that A$_3$AR activation appears to require flexibility at the 5'- and 3'-positions of the adenosine derivatives, which was diminished in both spiro and (N)-methanocarba analogues. In fact, MRS-1292 (**62**), which is a spiro adenosine derivative containing a 4',5'-lactam group, is a potent A$_3$ antagonist both in human (hA$_3$ K$_i$=29.3 nM) and rat (rA$_3$ K$_i$=51 nM) A$_3$ARs [296].

In preclinical tests, MRS-1292 (**62**) inhibits A$_3$AR-mediated shrinkage of human nonpigmented ciliary epithelial cells and reduces mouse intraocular pressure, supporting the potential use of A$_3$AR antagonists in glaucoma treatment [205]. Even a second alkylation at the nitrogen of the uronamido moiety at the 5' position of both adenosine and 4'-thioadenosine analogues, lead to the conversion of agonists in antagonists. In fact, MRS-3771 (**63**), the N,N-dimethyl analogue of Cl-IB-MECA (**4**), and LJ-1251 (**64**), the corresponding 4'-thio analogue, show competitive antagonism at the hA$_3$AR with affinity values of 29 nM and 15.5 nM, respectively [364]. Finally, similar results were obtained by complete removal of substituent at 4' position both in adenosine, 4'-thioadenosine and bicyclo[3.1.0]hexane derivatives [365].

LJ-1888 (**65**), belonging to the class of truncated 4'-thioadenosines, has been studied at preclinical level. One study reveals that LJ-1888 (**65**) induces anti-proliferation and apoptotic effects, via ERK and JNK activation, in T24 human bladder cancer cells, suggesting its use as an anticancer agent [238]. Another study on an unilateral ureteral obstruction rat model, shows that LJ-1888 (**65**) blocks the development of tubulointerstitial fibrosis and attenuated the progression of renal interstitial fibrosis [366]. MRS-5127 (**66**), MRS-5147 (**67**) and compound **68** are examples of A$_3$AR antagonists based on (N)-methanocarba structure [303, 367]. MRS-5127 (**66**) is an analogue of the agonist Cl-IB-MECA (**4**) and MRS-5147 (**67**) is its 3-bromo-benzyl derivative, whereas compound **68** is the corresponding antagonist of HEMADO (**7**). All these compounds show high affinity at the A$_3$AR (in both human and rat species).

Curiously, when stimulation of [^{35}S]GTPγS binding was used as a criterion of the hA$_3$AR receptor activation, MRS-5127 (**66**) and MRS-5147 (**67**) resulted antagonists (% efficacy < 10% of the full agonist NECA); whereas when the inhibition of the production of cAMP was measured, compounds showed a partial agonist behaviour (% efficacy 44-46% of the full agonist NECA) [300]. MRS-5127 (**66**) and MRS-5147 (**67**) were radiolabeled with ^{125}I and ^{76}Br, respectively, for their use as radioligands in pharmacologically receptor characterization (i.e., MRS-5127, **66**) [368] or as potential radiotracers for positron emission tomography (i.e., MRS-5147, **67**) [369]. Compound **68** demonstrated to be a potential protective agent for renal fibrosis in *in vitro* studies on mouse proximal tubular epithelial cells [367]. Finally, Santaris Pharma A/S has developed locked nucleosides based on the bicyclo[2.2.1]heptane scaffold and, among these derivatives, SPN-0234 (**69**) displays an IC$_{50}$ value of 8.2 nM at the hA$_3$AR, whereas it is completely inactive at the A$_1$ subtype [370].

There are some examples of adenosine derivatives bearing an intact ribose which displays antagonistic activity at the hA$_3$AR. Cosyn et al. synthesized 2-(1, 2, 3-triazolyl)adenosine derivatives bearing the ethyluronamido moiety or the natural hydroxyl group at the 5' position of the ribose ring.

Interestingly, several 5'-OH derivatives behave as antagonists, such as LC-153 (**70**); whereas the corresponding 5'-ethyluronamido derivatives are agonists or partial agonists. In 2006, Koch et al. of the Solvay Pharmaceuticals patented a series of 2-substituted-6-trifluoromethyl purine derivatives. All the reported compounds are A$_3$AR antagonists and one of the most representative derivatives is compound **71**, which bears a phenylethylamino moiety at the 2 position (hA$_3$ K$_i$=31.6 nM) (Figure 11, Table 6).

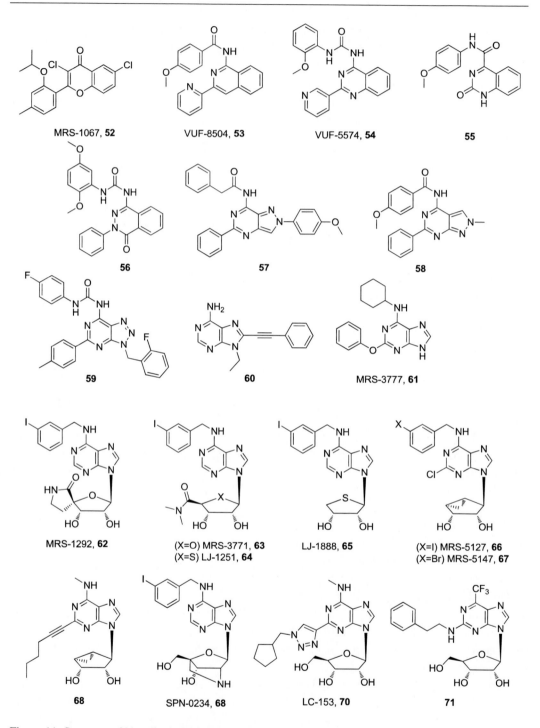

Figure 11. Structure of bicyclic A₃AR antagonists.

Table 6. Binding affinities of the bicyclic A$_3$AR antagonists at the A$_1$, A$_{2A}$, A$_{2B}$ and A$_3$ ARs

Compound	A$_1$ AR K$_i$ (nM) or % of displ.[a]	A$_{2A}$ AR K$_i$ (nM) or % of displ.[a]	A$_{2B}$ AR IC$_{50}$ (nM) or % of inhib.[b]	A$_3$ AR K$_i$ (nM)[c]	A$_1$/A$_3$	A$_{2A}$/A$_3$
52, MRS-1067 [346]	(r) 36% (100 μM)	(r) 19% (100 μM)	n.d.	561 (r) 5,500[d]	-	-
53, VUF-8504 [352]	(r) 14% (10 μM)	(r) 0% (10 μM)	n.d.	17	-	-
54, VUF-5574 [353]	(r) 52% (10 μM)	(r) 43% (10 μM)	n.d.	4.03	-	-
55 [355]	4% (1 μM)	1% (1 μM)	1% (1 μM)	19.5	> 51.3	> 51.3
56 [356]	0% (10 μM)	19% (10 μM)	0% (10 μM)	0.776	> 12,887	> 12,887
57 [358]	29% (1 μM)	18% (1 μM)	2% (1 μM)	24 (r) 3% (1 μM)	> 41.7	> 41.7
58 [359]	1,037	3,179	53.9	0.18	5,761	17,661
59 [360]	430	8,050	n.d.	6	72	1,342
60 [362]	1,300 (r) 2,600	600 (r) 640	≥ 30,000[e]	86 (r) 250	15 (r) 10.4	7 (r) 2.6
61, MRS-3777 [363]	26% (10 μM)	16% (10 μM)	13% (10 μM)	47	> 213	> 213
62, MRS-1292 [205, 296]	> 10,000 (r) 12,100	> 10,000 (r) 20,800	n.d.	29.3 (r) 51	> 341 (r) 237	>341 (r) 408
63 [364]	5,870	> 10,000	> 10,000	29	202	> 345
64 [364]	6,220	> 10,000	> 10,000	15.5	401	> 645
65 [365]	2,490	341	n.d.	4.16	599	82
66, MRS-5127 [298]	3,040	1,080	n.d.	1.44	2,111	750
67, MRS-5147 [298]	1,760	1,600	n.d.	0.73	2,411	2,192
68 [367]	14% (10 μM)	7,490	n.d.	4.90 (r) 231	> 2,041	1,529
69, SPN-0234 [370]	> 3,000[f]	n.d.	n.d.	8.2[f]	> 366	-
70, LC-153 [282]	335	39% (10 μM)	n.d.	1.3	258	> 7,692
71 [patent]	> 10,000	> 10,000	> 10,000[e]	31.6	> 316	> 316

[a] Displacement of specific radioligand binding, unless noted, in human ARs, expressed as K$_i$ values or % of displacement. A percent value indicates the percent displacement of radioligand at the concentration given in parentheses. (b): bovine; (r): rat. [b]Potency of examined compounds to inhibit stimulation of cAMP levels (cAMP assay) in CHO cells expressing hA$_{2B}$ARs, expressed as IC$_{50}$. A percent value indicates the percent inhibition of stimulated cAMP levels at the concentration given in parentheses. [c]Displacement of specific radioligand binding, unless noted, in human ARs, expressed as K$_i$ values. (r): rat.[d]for rat a functional cAMP assay was used. [e]K$_i$ value [f]IC$_{50}$ values.

Monocyclic Derivatives

1,4-Dihydropyridines bind to different targets of interest for medicinal chemistry (e.g., nifedipine is an L-type calcium channel inhibitor). Because certain 1,4-dihydropyridines were found to antagonize the A$_1$AR, Jacobson and co. decided to investigate 1,4-dihydropyridine derivatives for affinity at the A$_3$AR subtype [371]. In 1997, the first series of highly selective A$_3$ adenosine receptor antagonists bearing the 4-(phenylethynyl)-6-phenyl-1,4-dihydropyridine nucleus was reported [372]. MRS-1334 (**72**) belongs to this series, shows a K$_i$ of 2.69 nM at the hA$_3$AR and is more than 37'000 times selective *versus* the other AR subtypes. The same research group has explored even the pyridine scaffold [373]. The hybridization of the carbon at the 4 position of pyridine and 1,4-dihydropyridine, which is sp^2 and sp^3, respectively, confers a different steric control around this position in the two series. In fact, bulky 4-phenylethynyl moieties are tolerated in 1,4-dihydropyridines but not at the 4 position of the pyridine nucleus, which instead tolerates small alkyl groups. The pyridine compound MRS-1523 (73) bears a propyl group at the 4 position and displays affinity in the nanomolar range at both human (K_i=18.9 nM) and rat (K_i=113 nM) A_3ARs [373].

Also pyrimidines have been reported as A_3AR antagonists. Cosimelli et al. developed a series of 2-mercaptopyrimidines [374], whereas Yaziji et al. studied 2,6-diarylpyrimidines derivatives [375]. Compound 74 and ISVY-133 (75) are the most representative compounds of these series and show good affinity and selectivity profiles at the A_3AR (74, K_i = 3.5 nM; ISVY-133 75, K_i = 4.4 nM) (Figure 12, Table 7).

Finally, among 5-membered rings, thiadiazoles and thiazoles have been reported as potential potent and selective hA_3 antagonists [376]. A SAR study combined with molecular modeling approaches lead to the discovery of compound 76, a [1, 2, 4]thiadiazole displaying subnanomolar affinity at hA_3AR (K_i = 0.79 nM) and high subtype selectivity. Instead, the regioisomer N-(2-(4-methoxyphenyl)-[1, 3, 4]thiadiazol-5-yl)-acetamide shows only micromolar affinity at the hA_3AR. Molecular modeling studies demonstrated that contrary to that observed for compound 76, in the case of the [1, 3, 4]thiadiazole analogue, there was no H-bonding in its complex when docked in the hA_3AR binding cleft, supporting a more favourable binding pose for compound 76 than for its regioisomer [376].

Table 7. Binding affinities of the monocyclic A_3AR antagonists at the A_1, A_{2A}, A_{2B} and A_3 ARs

Compound	A_1 AR K_i (nM) or % of displ.[a]	A_{2A} AR K_i (nM) or % of displ.[a]	A_{2B} AR IC_{50} (nM) or % of displ.[b]	A_3 AR K_i (nM)[c]	A_1/A_3	A_{2A}/A_3
72, MRS-1334 [372]	(r) 29% (100 µM)	(r) < 10% (100 µM)	n.d.	2.69 (r) 3,850	-	-
73, MRS-1523 [373]	(r) 15,600	(r) 2,050	n.d.	18.9 (r) 113	(r) 138	(r) 18.1
74 [374]	17% (10 µM)	43% (10 µM)	> 10,000	3.5	> 2,857	> 2,857
75, ISVY-113 [375]	2% (0.1 µM)	8% (0.1 µM)	2% (0.1 µM)[d]	4.4	> 22.7	> 22.7
76 [376]	24% (10 µM)	28% (10 µM)	n.d.	0.79	> 12,658	> 12,658
77 [377]	> 10,000	> 10,000	3,200[e]	0.4	> 25,000	> 25,000
78 [378]	> 666	> 826	n.d.	0.36 (r) 1.6	5,761	17,661

[a] Displacement of specific radioligand binding, unless noted, in human ARs, expressed as K_i values or % of displacement. A percent value indicates the percent displacement of radioligand at the concentration given in parentheses. (b): bovine; (r): rat. [b] Potency of examined compounds to inhibit stimulation of cAMP levels (cAMP assay) in CHO cells expressing hA_{2B}ARs, expressed as IC_{50}. A percent value indicates the percent inhibition of stimulated cAMP levels at the concentration given in parentheses. [c] Displacement of specific radioligand binding, unless noted, in human ARs, expressed as K_i values. (r): rat. [d] Percentage of displacement of specific [³H]DPCPX binding at a concentration of 0.1 µM (n=2) in human HEK-293 cells. [e] K_b value.

At the same time, Novartis identified a class of potent, selective adenosine A$_3$ receptor antagonists, via optimisation of a screening hit thiazolic compound [377]. Structural modifications of the hit compound revealed that a pyridin-4-yl moiety at the 5 position of the thiazole ring was beneficial in terms of affinity at the A$_3$AR. Compound **77** is a highly potent hA$_3$AR antagonist with greater than 100-fold selectivity against the other AR subtypes and it also demonstrated to block the rat A$_3$ AR in *in vivo* studies [377].

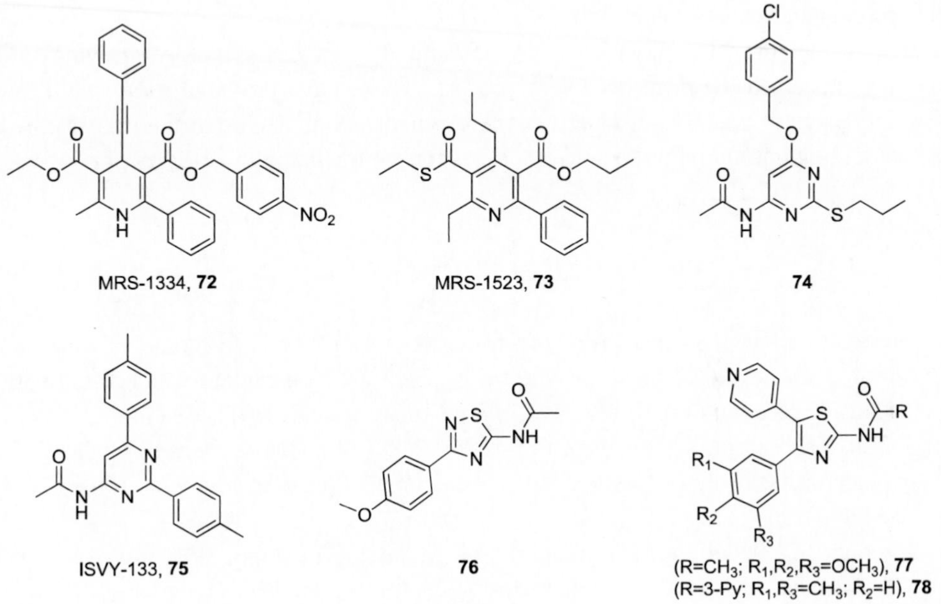

MRS-1334, **72**   MRS-1523, **73**   **74**

ISVY-133, **75**   **76**   (R=CH$_3$; R$_1$,R$_2$,R$_3$=OCH$_3$), **77**
(R=3-Py; R$_1$,R$_3$=CH$_3$; R$_2$=H), **78**

Figure 12. Structure of monocyclic A$_3$AR antagonists.

Takeda Pharmaceuticals further investigated this class of derivatives in order to develop an A$_3$AR antagonist with equipotent affinity and selectivity in human and rat, useful to evaluate its potential as a therapeutic target in asthma [378] (Figure 12, Table 7). The selected compound **79** inhibited IB-MECA-induced plasma protein extravasation in the skin of rats, and showed good oral absorption in rats. In addition, compound **79** significantly inhibited antigen-induced hyper-responsiveness to acetylcholine in actively sensitized Brown Norway rats, suggesting its usefulness as anti-asthmatic drug [378].

CONCLUSION

The A$_3$AR is a physiologically important therapeutic target as indicated by its potential pharmacological roles in our body. This receptor subtype has been shown to be involved in the pathophysiology of diseases through its modulation of pertinent signaling pathways. These biological functions and therapeutic applications of A$_3$AR have spurred the progress of development and identification of potent and selective A$_3$AR agonists and antagonists to tackle diseases of interest. This represents a preliminary stage towards wider clinical applications of ligands selective against this still enigmatic receptor. Nonetheless, it has paved the way for a clearer understanding of clinical relevance of this receptor in many pathophysiological conditions, such as inflammatory disorders and cancer. Specifically, the role of A_3AR in regulating inflammatory and immune responses evince its therapeutic significance for inflammatory conditions such as asthma, rheumatoid arthritis and psoriasis. This is reflected in promising clinical data obtained for certain A_3AR agonists as potential antirheumatic drugs. Moreover, A_3AR agonist Cl-IB-MECA has been shown efficacious in several animal tumor models in preclinical trials. Consistently, it demonstrates good safety profile in Phase I clinical trials, and currently undergoes Phase II clinical studies in patients with hepatocellular carcinoma.

As a whole, the investigations of A_3AR and its ligands is rapidly growing with an increasing impact on the drug discovery process. These have provided useful path towards successful design of potent and selective A_3AR ligands which can be further transformed into drugs possessing optimum therapeutic outcomes for the treatment of diseases of concern.

REFERENCES

[1] Fredholm, BB; IJzerman, AP; Jacobson, KA; Linden, J; Muller, CE. International Union of Basic and Clinical Pharmacology. LXXXI. Nomenclature and classification of adenosine receptors--an update. *Pharmacological reviews*, 2011, 63 (1), 1-34.

[2] Borea, PA; Varani, K; Vincenzi, F; Baraldi, PG; Tabrizi, MA; Merighi, S; Gessi, S. The A3 adenosine receptor: history and perspectives. *Pharmacological reviews*, 2015, 67 (1), 74-102.

[3] Cheong, SL; Federico, S; Venkatesan, G; Mandel, AL; Shao, YM; Moro, S; Spalluto, G; Pastorin, G. The A3 adenosine receptor as multifaceted therapeutic target: pharmacology, medicinal chemistry, and in silico approaches. *Medicinal research reviews*, 2013, 33 (2), 235-335.

[4] Meyerhof, W; Muller-Brechlin, R; Richter, D. Molecular cloning of a novel putative G-protein coupled receptor expressed during rat spermiogenesis. *FEBS letters*, 1991, 284 (2), 155-60.

[5] Zhou, QY; Li, C; Olah, ME; Johnson, RA; Stiles, GL; Civelli, O. Molecular cloning and characterization of an adenosine receptor: the A3 adenosine receptor. *Proceedings of the National Academy of Sciences of the United States of America*, 1992, 89 (16), 7432-6.

[6] Linden, J. Cloned adenosine A3 receptors: pharmacological properties, species differences and receptor functions. *Trends in pharmacological sciences*, 1994, 15 (8), 298-306.

[7] Jacobson, KA; Gao, ZG. Adenosine receptors as therapeutic targets. *Nature reviews. Drug discovery*, 2006, 5 (3), 247-64.

[8] Murrison, EM; Goodson, SJ; Edbrooke, MR; Harris, CA. Cloning and characterisation of the human adenosine A3 receptor gene. *FEBS letters*, 1996, 384 (3), 243-6.

[9] Yamano, K; Inoue, M; Masaki, S; Saki, M; Ichimura, M; Satoh, M. Generation of adenosine A3 receptor functionally humanized mice for the evaluation of the human antagonists. *Biochemical pharmacology*, 2006, 71 (3), 294-306.

[10] Atkinson, MR; Townsend-Nicholson, A; Nicholl, JK; Sutherland, GR; Schofield, PR. Cloning, characterisation and chromosomal assignment of the human adenosine A3 receptor (ADORA3) gene. *Neuroscience research*, 1997, 29 (1), 73-9.

[11] Gilman, AG. G proteins: transducers of receptor-generated signals. *Annual review of biochemistry*, 1987, 56, 615-49.

[12] Kim, SK; Gao, ZG; Van Rompaey, P; Gross, AS; Chen, A; Van Calenbergh, S; Jacobson, KA. Modeling the adenosine receptors: comparison of the binding domains of A2A agonists and antagonists. *Journal of medicinal chemistry*, 2003, 46 (23), 4847-59.

[13] Palmer, TM; Benovic, JL; Stiles, GL. Agonist-dependent phosphorylation and desensitization of the rat A3 adenosine receptor. Evidence for a G-protein-coupled receptor kinase-mediated mechanism. *The Journal of biological chemistry*, 1995, 270 (49), 29607-13.

[14] Trincavelli, ML; Tuscano, D; Marroni, M; Falleni, A; Gremigni, V; Ceruti, S; Abbracchio, MP; Jacobson, KA; Cattabeni, F; Martini, C. A3 adenosine receptors in human astrocytoma cells: agonist-mediated desensitization, internalization, and down-regulation. *Molecular pharmacology*, 2002, 62 (6), 1373-84.

[15] Madi, L; Bar-Yehuda, S; Barer, F; Ardon, E; Ochaion, A; Fishman, P. A3 adenosine receptor activation in melanoma cells: association between receptor fate and tumor growth inhibition. *The Journal of biological chemistry*, 2003, 278 (43), 42121-30.

[16] May, LT; Bridge, LJ; Stoddart, LA; Briddon, SJ; Hill, SJ. Allosteric interactions across native adenosine-A3 receptor homodimers: quantification using single-cell ligand-binding kinetics. *FASEB journal : official publication of the Federation of American Societies for Experimental Biology*, 2011, 25 (10), 3465-76.

[17] Kim, SK; Jacobson, KA. Computational prediction of homodimerization of the A3 adenosine receptor. *Journal of molecular graphics & modelling*, 2006, 25 (4), 549-61.

[18] Merighi, S; Mirandola, P; Varani, K; Gessi, S; Leung, E; Baraldi, PG; Tabrizi, MA; Borea, PA. A glance at adenosine receptors: novel target for antitumor therapy. *Pharmacology & therapeutics*, 2003, 100 (1), 31-48.

[19] Ali, H; Cunha-Melo, JR; Saul, WF; Beaven, MA. Activation of phospholipase C via adenosine receptors provides synergistic signals for secretion in antigen-stimulated RBL-2H3 cells. Evidence for a novel adenosine receptor. *The Journal of biological chemistry*, 1990, 265 (2), 745-53.

[20] Abbracchio, MP; Brambilla, R; Ceruti, S; Kim, HO; von Lubitz, DK; Jacobson, KA; Cattabeni, F. G protein-dependent activation of phospholipase C by adenosine A3 receptors in rat brain. *Molecular pharmacology*, 1995, 48 (6), 1038-45.

[21] Mozzicato, S; Joshi, BV; Jacobson, KA; Liang, BT. Role of direct RhoA-phospholipase D1 interaction in mediating adenosine-induced protection from cardiac ischemia. *FASEB journal : official publication of the Federation of American Societies for Experimental Biology*, 2004, 18 (2), 406-8.

[22] Tracey, WR; Magee, W; Masamune, H; Oleynek, JJ; Hill, RJ. Selective activation of adenosine A3 receptors with N6-(3-chlorobenzyl)-5'-N-methylcarboxamidoadenosine (CB-MECA) provides cardioprotection via KATP channel activation. *Cardiovascular research*, 1998, 40 (1), 138-45.

[23] Wan, TC; Ge, ZD; Tampo, A; Mio, Y; Bienengraeber, MW; Tracey, WR; Gross, GJ; Kwok, WM; Auchampach, JA. The A3 adenosine receptor agonist CP-532,903 [N6-

(2,5-dichlorobenzyl)-3'-aminoadenosine-5'-N-methylcarboxamide] protects against myocardial ischemia/reperfusion injury via the sarcolemmal ATP-sensitive potassium channel. *The Journal of pharmacology and experimental therapeutics*, 2008, 324 (1), 234-43.

[24] Schulte, G; Fredholm, BB. Human adenosine A(1), A(2A), A(2B), and A(3) receptors expressed in Chinese hamster ovary cells all mediate the phosphorylation of extracellular-regulated kinase 1/2. *Molecular pharmacology*, 2000, 58 (3), 477-82.

[25] Schulte, G; Fredholm, BB. Signaling pathway from the human adenosine A(3) receptor expressed in Chinese hamster ovary cells to the extracellular signal-regulated kinase 1/2. *Molecular pharmacology*, 2002, 62 (5), 1137-46.

[26] Hammarberg, C; Schulte, G; Fredholm, BB. Evidence for functional adenosine A3 receptors in microglia cells. *Journal of neurochemistry*, 2003, 86 (4), 1051-4.

[27] Merighi, S; Benini, A; Mirandola, P; Gessi, S; Varani, K; Leung, E; Maclennan, S; Baraldi, PG; Borea, PA. Hypoxia inhibits paclitaxel-induced apoptosis through adenosine-mediated phosphorylation of bad in glioblastoma cells. *Molecular pharmacology*, 2007, 72 (1), 162-72.

[28] Merighi, S; Mirandola, P; Milani, D; Varani, K; Gessi, S; Klotz, KN; Leung, E; Baraldi, PG; Borea, PA. Adenosine receptors as mediators of both cell proliferation and cell death of cultured human melanoma cells. *The Journal of investigative dermatology*, 2002, 119 (4), 923-33.

[29] Germack, R; Dickenson, JM. Adenosine triggers preconditioning through MEK/ERK1/2 signalling pathway during hypoxia/ reoxygenation in neonatal rat cardiomyocytes. *Journal of molecular and cellular cardiology*, 2005, 39 (3), 429-42.

[30] Germack, R; Dickenson, JM. Characterization of ERK1/2 signalling pathways induced by adenosine receptor subtypes in newborn rat cardiomyocytes. *British journal of pharmacology*, 2004, 141 (2), 329-39.

[31] Salie, R; Moolman, JA; Lochner, A. The mechanism of beta-adrenergic preconditioning: roles for adenosine and ROS during triggering and mediation. *Basic research in cardiology*, 2012, 107 (5), 281.

[32] Gessi, S; Sacchetto, V; Fogli, E; Merighi, S; Varani, K; Baraldi, PG; Tabrizi, MA; Leung, E; Maclennan, S; Borea, PA. Modulation of metalloproteinase-9 in U87MG glioblastoma cells by A3 adenosine receptors. *Biochemical pharmacology*, 2010, 79 (10), 1483-95.

[33] Hasko, G; Nemeth, ZH; Vizi, ES; Salzman, AL; Szabo, C. An agonist of adenosine A3 receptors decreases interleukin-12 and interferon-gamma production and prevents lethality in endotoxemic mice. *European journal of pharmacology*, 1998, 358 (3), 261-8.

[34] Lee, HS; Chung, HJ; Lee, HW; Jeong, LS; Lee, SK. Suppression of inflammation response by a novel A(3) adenosine receptor agonist thio-Cl-IB-MECA through inhibition of Akt and NF-kappaB signaling. *Immunobiology*, 2011, 216 (9), 997-1003.

[35] Lee, JY; Jhun, BS; Oh, YT; Lee, JH; Choe, W; Baik, HH; Ha, J; Yoon, KS; Kim, SS; Kang, I. Activation of adenosine A3 receptor suppresses lipopolysaccharide-induced TNF-alpha production through inhibition of PI 3-kinase/Akt and NF-kappaB activation in murine BV2 microglial cells. *Neuroscience letters*, 2006, 396 (1), 1-6.

[36] Linden, J; Taylor, HE; Robeva, AS; Tucker, AL; Stehle, JH; Rivkees, SA; Fink, JS; Reppert, SM. Molecular cloning and functional expression of a sheep A3 adenosine

receptor with widespread tissue distribution. *Molecular pharmacology*, 1993, 44 (3), 524-32.

[37] Salvatore, CA; Jacobson, MA; Taylor, HE; Linden, J; Johnson, RG. Molecular cloning and characterization of the human A3 adenosine receptor. *Proceedings of the National Academy of Sciences of the United States of America*, 1993, 90 (21), 10365-9.

[38] Ramkumar, V; Stiles, GL; Beaven, MA; Ali, H. The A3 adenosine receptor is the unique adenosine receptor which facilitates release of allergic mediators in mast cells. *The Journal of biological chemistry*, 1993, 268 (23), 16887-90.

[39] Hannon, JP; Pfannkuche, HJ; Fozard, JR. A role for mast cells in adenosine A3 receptor-mediated hypotension in the rat. *British journal of pharmacology*, 1995, 115 (6), 945-52.

[40] Fozard, JR; Pfannkuche, HJ; Schuurman, HJ. Mast cell degranulation following adenosine A3 receptor activation in rats. *European journal of pharmacology*, 1996, 298 (3), 293-7.

[41] Leung, CT; Li, A; Banerjee, J; Gao, ZG; Kambayashi, T; Jacobson, KA; Civan, MM. The role of activated adenosine receptors in degranulation of human LAD2 mast cells. *Purinergic signalling*, 2014, 10 (3), 465-75.

[42] Kohno, Y; Ji, X; Mawhorter, SD; Koshiba, M; Jacobson, KA. Activation of A3 adenosine receptors on human eosinophils elevates intracellular calcium. *Blood*, 1996, 88 (9), 3569-74.

[43] Bouma, MG; Jeunhomme, TM; Boyle, DL; Dentener, MA; Voitenok, NN; van den Wildenberg, FA; Buurman, WA. Adenosine inhibits neutrophil degranulation in activated human whole blood: involvement of adenosine A2 and A3 receptors. *Journal of immunology*, 1997, 158 (11), 5400-8.

[44] Gessi, S; Varani, K; Merighi, S; Cattabriga, E; Iannotta, V; Leung, E; Baraldi, PG; Borea, PA. A(3) adenosine receptors in human neutrophils and promyelocytic HL60 cells: a pharmacological and biochemical study. *Molecular pharmacology*, 2002, 61 (2), 415-24.

[45] Thiele, A; Kronstein, R; Wetzel, A; Gerth, A; Nieber, K; Hauschildt, S. Regulation of adenosine receptor subtypes during cultivation of human monocytes: role of receptors in preventing lipopolysaccharide-triggered respiratory burst. *Infection and immunity*, 2004, 72 (3), 1349-57.

[46] Broussas, M; Cornillet-Lefebvre, P; Potron, G; Nguyen, P. Adenosine inhibits tissue factor expression by LPS-stimulated human monocytes: involvement of the A3 adenosine receptor. *Thrombosis and haemostasis*, 2002, 88 (1), 123-30.

[47] Szabo, C; Scott, GS; Virag, L; Egnaczyk, G; Salzman, AL; Shanley, TP; Hasko, G. Suppression of macrophage inflammatory protein (MIP)-1alpha production and collagen-induced arthritis by adenosine receptor agonists. *British journal of pharmacology*, 1998, 125 (2), 379-87.

[48] McWhinney, CD; Dudley, MW; Bowlin, TL; Peet, NP; Schook, L; Bradshaw, M; De, M; Borcherding, DR; Edwards, CK. 3rd, Activation of adenosine A3 receptors on macrophages inhibits tumor necrosis factor-alpha. *European journal of pharmacology*, 1996, 310 (2-3), 209-16.

[49] Fossetta, J; Jackson, J; Deno, G; Fan, X; Du, XK; Bober, L; Soude-Bermejo, A; de Bouteiller, O; Caux, C; Lunn, C; Lundell, D; Palmer, RK. Pharmacological analysis of

calcium responses mediated by the human A3 adenosine receptor in monocyte-derived dendritic cells and recombinant cells. *Molecular pharmacology*, 2003, 63 (2), 342-50.

[50] Hofer, S; Ivarsson, L; Stoitzner, P; Auffinger, M; Rainer, C; Romani, N; Heufler, C. Adenosine slows migration of dendritic cells but does not affect other aspects of dendritic cell maturation. *The Journal of investigative dermatology*, 2003, 121 (2), 300-7.

[51] Dickenson, JM; Reeder, S; Rees, B; Alexander, S; Kendall, D. Functional expression of adenosine A2A and A3 receptors in the mouse dendritic cell line XS-106. *European journal of pharmacology*, 2003, 474 (1), 43-51.

[52] Gessi, S; Varani, K; Merighi, S; Cattabriga, E; Avitabile, A; Gavioli, R; Fortini, C; Leung, E; Mac Lennan, S; Borea, PA. Expression of A3 adenosine receptors in human lymphocytes: up-regulation in T cell activation. *Molecular pharmacology*, 2004, 65 (3), 711-9.

[53] Suh, BC; Kim, TD; Lee, JU; Seong, JK; Kim, KT. Pharmacological characterization of adenosine receptors in PGT-beta mouse pineal gland tumour cells. *British journal of pharmacology*, 2001, 134 (1), 132-42.

[54] Merighi, S; Varani, K; Gessi, S; Cattabriga, E; Iannotta, V; Ulouglu, C; Leung, E; Borea, PA. Pharmacological and biochemical characterization of adenosine receptors in the human malignant melanoma A375 cell line. *British journal of pharmacology*, 2001, 134 (6), 1215-26.

[55] Gessi, S; Merighi, S; Varani, K; Cattabriga, E; Benini, A; Mirandola, P; Leung, E; Mac Lennan, S; Feo, C; Baraldi, S; Borea, PA. Adenosine receptors in colon carcinoma tissues and colon tumoral cell lines: focus on the A(3) adenosine subtype. *Journal of cellular physiology*, 2007, 211 (3), 826-36.

[56] Gessi, S; Varani, K; Merighi, S; Morelli, A; Ferrari, D; Leung, E; Baraldi, PG; Spalluto, G; Borea, PA. Pharmacological and biochemical characterization of A3 adenosine receptors in Jurkat T cells. *British journal of pharmacology*, 2001, 134 (1), 116-26.

[57] Madi, L; Cohen, S; Ochayin, A; Bar-Yehuda, S; Barer, F; Fishman, P. Overexpression of A3 adenosine receptor in peripheral blood mononuclear cells in rheumatoid arthritis: involvement of nuclear factor-kappaB in mediating receptor level. *The Journal of rheumatology*, 2007, 34 (1), 20-6.

[58] Madi, L; Ochaion, A; Rath-Wolfson, L; Bar-Yehuda, S; Erlanger, A; Ohana, G; Harish, A; Merimski, O; Barer, F; Fishman, P. The A3 adenosine receptor is highly expressed in tumor versus normal cells: potential target for tumor growth inhibition. *Clinical cancer research : an official journal of the American Association for Cancer Research*, 2004, 10 (13), 4472-9.

[59] Bar-Yehuda, S; Stemmer, S; Madi, L; Castel, D; Ochaion, A; Cohen, S; Barer, F; Zabutti, A; Perez-Liz, G; Del Valle, L. The A3 adenosine receptor agonist CF102 induces apoptosis of hepatocellular carcinoma via de-regulation of the Wnt and NF-κB signal transduction pathways. *International journal of oncology*, 2008, 33 (2), 287-295.

[60] Headrick, JP; Peart, JN; Reichelt, ME; Haseler, LJ. Adenosine and its receptors in the heart: regulation, retaliation and adaptation. *Biochimica et biophysica acta*, 2011, 1808 (5), 1413-28.

[61] Peart, JN; Headrick, JP. Adenosinergic cardioprotection: multiple receptors, multiple pathways. *Pharmacology & therapeutics*, 2007, 114 (2), 208-21.

[62] Tracey, WR; Magee, W; Masamune, H; Kennedy, SP; Knight, DR; Buchholz, RA; Hill, RJ. Selective adenosine A3 receptor stimulation reduces ischemic myocardial injury in the rabbit heart. *Cardiovascular research*, 1997, 33 (2), 410-5.

[63] Xu, Z; Jang, Y; Mueller, RA; Norfleet, EA. IB-MECA and cardioprotection. *Cardiovascular drug reviews*, 2006, 24 (3-4), 227-38.

[64] Jacobson, KA; Nikodijevic, O; Shi, D; Gallo-Rodriguez, C; Olah, ME; Stiles, GL; Daly, JW. A role for central A3-adenosine receptors. Mediation of behavioral depressant effects. *FEBS letters*, 1993, 336 (1), 57-60.

[65] Gessi, S; Merighi, S; Stefanelli, A; Fazzi, D; Varani, K; Borea, PA. A(1) and A(3) adenosine receptors inhibit LPS-induced hypoxia-inducible factor-1 accumulation in murine astrocytes. *Pharmacological research : the official journal of the Italian Pharmacological Society*, 2013, 76, 157-70.

[66] Ohsawa, K; Sanagi, T; Nakamura, Y; Suzuki, E; Inoue, K; Kohsaka, S. Adenosine A3 receptor is involved in ADP-induced microglial process extension and migration. *Journal of neurochemistry*, 2012, 121 (2), 217-27.

[67] Kobie, JJ; Shah, PR; Yang, L; Rebhahn, JA; Fowell, DJ; Mosmann, TR. T regulatory and primed uncommitted CD4 T cells express CD73, which suppresses effector CD4 T cells by converting 5'-adenosine monophosphate to adenosine. *Journal of immunology*, 2006, 177 (10), 6780-6.

[68] Deaglio, S; Dwyer, KM; Gao, W; Friedman, D; Usheva, A; Erat, A; Chen, JF; Enjyoji, K; Linden, J; Oukka, M; Kuchroo, VK; Strom, TB; Robson, SC. Adenosine generation catalyzed by CD39 and CD73 expressed on regulatory T cells mediates immune suppression. *The Journal of experimental medicine*, 2007, 204 (6), 1257-65.

[69] Zimmermann, H. Extracellular metabolism of ATP and other nucleotides. *Naunyn-Schmiedeberg's archives of pharmacology*, 2000, 362 (4-5), 299-309.

[70] Deussen, A. Metabolic flux rates of adenosine in the heart. *Naunyn-Schmiedeberg's archives of pharmacology*, 2000, 362 (4-5), 351-63.

[71] Kadl, A; Leitinger, N. The role of endothelial cells in the resolution of acute inflammation. *Antioxidants & redox signaling*, 2005, 7 (11-12), 1744-54.

[72] Mann, JS; Renwick, AG; Holgate, ST. Release of adenosine and its metabolites from activated human leucocytes. *Clinical science*, 1986, 70 (5), 461-8.

[73] Cronstein, BN; Kramer, SB; Weissmann, G; Hirschhorn, R. Adenosine: a physiological modulator of superoxide anion generation by human neutrophils. *The Journal of experimental medicine*, 1983, 158 (4), 1160-77.

[74] Madara, JL; Patapoff, TW; Gillece-Castro, B; Colgan, SP; Parkos, CA; Delp, C; Mrsny, RJ., 5'-adenosine monophosphate is the neutrophil-derived paracrine factor that elicits chloride secretion from T84 intestinal epithelial cell monolayers. *The Journal of clinical investigation*, 1993, 91 (5), 2320-5.

[75] Rounds, S; Hsieh, L; Agarwal, KC. Effects of endotoxin injury on endothelial cell adenosine metabolism. *The Journal of laboratory and clinical medicine*, 1994, 123 (2), 309-17.

[76] Fredholm, BB. Adenosine, an endogenous distress signal, modulates tissue damage and repair. *Cell death and differentiation*, 2007, 14 (7), 1315-23.

[77] Eppell, BA; Newell, AM; Brown, EJ. Adenosine receptors are expressed during differentiation of monocytes to macrophages in vitro. Implications for regulation of phagocytosis. *Journal of immunology*, 1989, 143 (12), 4141-5.

[78] Salmon, JE; Brogle, N; Brownlie, C; Edberg, JC; Kimberly, RP; Chen, BX; Erlanger, BF. Human mononuclear phagocytes express adenosine A1 receptors. A novel mechanism for differential regulation of Fc gamma receptor function. *Journal of immunology*, 1993, 151 (5), 2775-85.

[79] Clark, AN; Youkey, R; Liu, X; Jia, L; Blatt, R; Day, YJ; Sullivan, GW; Linden, J; Tucker, AL. A1 adenosine receptor activation promotes angiogenesis and release of VEGF from monocytes. *Circulation research*, 2007, 101 (11), 1130-8.

[80] Le Vraux, V; Chen, YL; Masson, I; De Sousa, M; Giroud, JP; Florentin, I; Chauvelot-Moachon, L. Inhibition of human monocyte TNF production by adenosine receptor agonists. *Life sciences*, 1993, 52 (24), 1917-24.

[81] Hasko, G; Szabo, C; Nemeth, ZH; Kvetan, V; Pastores, SM; Vizi, ES. Adenosine receptor agonists differentially regulate IL-10, TNF-alpha, and nitric oxide production in RAW 264.7 macrophages and in endotoxemic mice. *Journal of immunology*, 1996, 157 (10), 4634-40.

[82] Hasko, G; Kuhel, DG; Chen, JF; Schwarzschild, MA; Deitch, EA; Mabley, JG; Marton, A; Szabo, C. Adenosine inhibits IL-12 and TNF-[alpha] production via adenosine A2a receptor-dependent and independent mechanisms. *FASEB journal : official publication of the Federation of American Societies for Experimental Biology*, 2000, 14 (13), 2065-74.

[83] Hasko, G; Pacher, P; Deitch, EA; Vizi, ES. Shaping of monocyte and macrophage function by adenosine receptors. *Pharmacology & therapeutics*, 2007, 113 (2), 264-75.

[84] Link, AA; Kino, T; Worth, JA; McGuire, JL; Crane, ML; Chrousos, GP; Wilder, RL; Elenkov, IJ. Ligand-activation of the adenosine A2a receptors inhibits IL-12 production by human monocytes. *Journal of immunology*, 2000, 164 (1), 436-42.

[85] Khoa, ND; Montesinos, MC; Reiss, AB; Delano, D; Awadallah, N; Cronstein, BN. Inflammatory cytokines regulate function and expression of adenosine A(2A) receptors in human monocytic THP-1 cells. *Journal of immunology*, 2001, 167 (7), 4026-32.

[86] Nemeth, ZH; Lutz, CS; Csoka, B; Deitch, EA; Leibovich, SJ; Gause, WC; Tone, M; Pacher, P; Vizi, ES; Hasko, G. Adenosine augments IL-10 production by macrophages through an A2B receptor-mediated posttranscriptional mechanism. *Journal of immunology*, 2005, 175 (12), 8260-70.

[87] Zhang, JG; Hepburn, L; Cruz, G; Borman, RA; Clark, KL. The role of adenosine A2A and A2B receptors in the regulation of TNF-alpha production by human monocytes. *Biochemical pharmacology*, 2005, 69 (6), 883-9.

[88] la Sala, A; Gadina, M; Kelsall, BL. G(i)-protein-dependent inhibition of IL-12 production is mediated by activation of the phosphatidylinositol 3-kinase-protein 3 kinase B/Akt pathway and JNK. *Journal of immunology*, 2005, 175 (5), 2994-9.

[89] Marone, G; Petracca, R; Vigorita, S; Genovese, A; Casolaro, V. Adenosine receptors on human leukocytes. IV. Characterization of an A1/Ri receptor. *International journal of clinical & laboratory research*, 1992, 22 (4), 235-42.

[90] Fortin, A; Harbour, D; Fernandes, M; Borgeat, P; Bourgoin, S. Differential expression of adenosine receptors in human neutrophils: up-regulation by specific Th1 cytokines and lipopolysaccharide. *Journal of leukocyte biology*, 2006, 79 (3), 574-85.

[91] Bours, MJ; Swennen, EL; Di Virgilio, F; Cronstein, BN; Dagnelie, PC. Adenosine 5'-triphosphate and adenosine as endogenous signaling molecules in immunity and inflammation. *Pharmacology & therapeutics*, 2006, 112 (2), 358-404.

[92] Cronstein, BN; Daguma, L; Nichols, D; Hutchison, AJ; Williams, M. The adenosine/neutrophil paradox resolved: human neutrophils possess both A1 and A2 receptors that promote chemotaxis and inhibit O2 generation, respectively. *The Journal of clinical investigation*, 1990, 85 (4), 1150-7.

[93] Salmon, JE; Cronstein, BN. Fc gamma receptor-mediated functions in neutrophils are modulated by adenosine receptor occupancy. A1 receptors are stimulatory and A2 receptors are inhibitory. *Journal of immunology*, 1990, 145 (7), 2235-40.

[94] Sullivan, GW; Lee, DD; Ross, WG; DiVietro, JA; Lappas, CM; Lawrence, MB; Linden, J. Activation of A2A adenosine receptors inhibits expression of alpha 4/beta 1 integrin (very late antigen-4) on stimulated human neutrophils. *Journal of leukocyte biology*, 2004, 75 (1), 127-34.

[95] McPherson, JA; Barringhaus, KG; Bishop, GG; Sanders, JM; Rieger, JM; Hesselbacher, SE; Gimple, LW; Powers, ER; Macdonald, T; Sullivan, G; Linden, J; Sarembock, IJ. Adenosine A(2A) receptor stimulation reduces inflammation and neointimal growth in a murine carotid ligation model. *Arteriosclerosis, thrombosis, and vascular biology*, 2001, 21 (5), 791-6.

[96] Flamand, N; Lefebvre, J; Lapointe, G; Picard, S; Lemieux, L; Bourgoin, SG; Borgeat, P. Inhibition of platelet-activating factor biosynthesis by adenosine and histamine in human neutrophils: involvement of cPLA2alpha and reversal by lyso-PAF. *Journal of leukocyte biology*, 2006, 79 (5), 1043-51.

[97] Flamand, N; Boudreault, S; Picard, S; Austin, M; Surette, ME; Plante, H; Krump, E; Vallee, MJ; Gilbert, C; Naccache, P; Laviolette, M; Borgeat, P. Adenosine, a potent natural suppressor of arachidonic acid release and leukotriene biosynthesis in human neutrophils. *American journal of respiratory and critical care medicine*, 2000, 161 (2 Pt 2), S88-94.

[98] Flamand, N; Surette, ME; Picard, S; Bourgoin, S; Borgeat, P. Cyclic AMP-mediated inhibition of 5-lipoxygenase translocation and leukotriene biosynthesis in human neutrophils. *Molecular pharmacology*, 2002, 62 (2), 250-6.

[99] Grenier, S; Flamand, N; Pelletier, J; Naccache, PH; Borgeat, P; Bourgoin, SG. Arachidonic acid activates phospholipase D in human neutrophils; essential role of endogenous leukotriene B4 and inhibition by adenosine A2A receptor engagement. *Journal of leukocyte biology*, 2003, 73 (4), 530-9.

[100] Krump, E; Lemay, G; Borgeat, P. Adenosine A2 receptor-induced inhibition of leukotriene B4 synthesis in whole blood ex vivo. *British journal of pharmacology*, 1996, 117 (8), 1639-44.

[101] Krump, E; Picard, S; Mancini, J; Borgeat, P. Suppression of leukotriene B4 biosynthesis by endogenous adenosine in ligand-activated human neutrophils. *The Journal of experimental medicine*, 1997, 186 (8), 1401-6.

[102] Krump, E; Borgeat, P. Adenosine. An endogenous inhibitor of arachidonic acid release and leukotriene biosynthesis in human neutrophils. *Advances in experimental medicine and biology*, 1999, 447, 107-15.

[103] Surette, ME; Krump, E; Picard, S; Borgeat, P. Activation of leukotriene synthesis in human neutrophils by exogenous arachidonic acid: inhibition by adenosine A(2a) receptor agonists and crucial role of autocrine activation by leukotriene B(4). *Molecular pharmacology*, 1999, 56 (5), 1055-62.

[104] Wakai, A; Wang, JH; Winter, DC; Street, JT; O'Sullivan, RG; Redmond, HP. Adenosine inhibits neutrophil vascular endothelial growth factor release and transendothelial migration via A2B receptor activation. *Shock*, 2001, 15 (4), 297-301.

[105] Fishman, P; Bar-Yehuda, S. Pharmacology and therapeutic applications of A3 receptor subtype. *Current topics in medicinal chemistry*, 2003, 3 (4), 463-9.

[106] Walker, BA; Jacobson, MA; Knight, DA; Salvatore, CA; Weir, T; Zhou, D; Bai, TR. Adenosine A3 receptor expression and function in eosinophils. *American journal of respiratory cell and molecular biology*, 1997, 16 (5), 531-7.

[107] Ezeamuzie, CI; Philips, E. Adenosine A3 receptors on human eosinophils mediate inhibition of degranulation and superoxide anion release. *British journal of pharmacology*, 1999, 127 (1), 188-94.

[108] Knight, D; Zheng, X; Rocchini, C; Jacobson, M; Bai, T; Walker, B. Adenosine A3 receptor stimulation inhibits migration of human eosinophils. *Journal of leukocyte biology*, 1997, 62 (4), 465-8.

[109] Salvatore, CA; Tilley, SL; Latour, AM; Fletcher, DS; Koller, BH; Jacobson, MA. Disruption of the A(3) adenosine receptor gene in mice and its effect on stimulated inflammatory cells. *The Journal of biological chemistry*, 2000, 275 (6), 4429-34.

[110] Zhong, H; Shlykov, SG; Molina, JG; Sanborn, BM; Jacobson, MA; Tilley, SL; Blackburn, MR. Activation of murine lung mast cells by the adenosine A3 receptor. *Journal of immunology*, 2003, 171 (1), 338-45.

[111] Feoktistov, I; Biaggioni, I. Adenosine A2b receptors evoke interleukin-8 secretion in human mast cells. An enprofylline-sensitive mechanism with implications for asthma. *The Journal of clinical investigation*, 1995, 96 (4), 1979-86.

[112] Ryzhov, S; Goldstein, AE; Matafonov, A; Zeng, D; Biaggioni, I; Feoktistov, I. Adenosine-activated mast cells induce IgE synthesis by B lymphocytes: an A2B-mediated process involving Th2 cytokines IL-4 and IL-13 with implications for asthma. *Journal of immunology*, 2004, 172 (12), 7726-33.

[113] Ryzhov, S; Zaynagetdinov, R; Goldstein, AE; Novitskiy, SV; Dikov, MM; Blackburn, MR; Biaggioni, I; Feoktistov, I. Effect of A2B adenosine receptor gene ablation on proinflammatory adenosine signaling in mast cells. *Journal of immunology*, 2008, 180 (11), 7212-20.

[114] Marone, G; Vigorita, S; Triggiani, M; Condorelli, M. Adenosine receptors on human lymphocytes. *Advances in experimental medicine and biology*, 1986, 195 *Pt B*, 7-14.

[115] Huang, S; Apasov, S; Koshiba, M; Sitkovsky, M. Role of A2a extracellular adenosine receptor-mediated signaling in adenosine-mediated inhibition of T-cell activation and expansion. *Blood*, 1997, 90 (4), 1600-10.

[116] Mirabet, M; Mallol, J; Lluis, C; Franco, R. Calcium mobilization in Jurkat cells via A2b adenosine receptors. *British journal of pharmacology*, 1997, 122 (6), 1075-82.

[117] Koshiba, M; Kojima, H; Huang, S; Apasov, S; Sitkovsky, MV. Memory of extracellular adenosine A2A purinergic receptor-mediated signaling in murine T cells. *The Journal of biological chemistry*, 1997, 272 (41), 25881-9.

[118] Koshiba, M; Rosin, DL; Hayashi, N; Linden, J; Sitkovsky, MV. Patterns of A2A extracellular adenosine receptor expression in different functional subsets of human peripheral T cells. Flow cytometry studies with anti-A2A receptor monoclonal antibodies. *Molecular pharmacology*, 1999, 55 (3), 614-24.

[119] Hoskin, DW; Mader, JS; Furlong, SJ; Conrad, DM; Blay, J. Inhibition of T cell and natural killer cell function by adenosine and its contribution to immune evasion by tumor cells (Review). *International journal of oncology*, 2008, 32 (3), 527-35.

[120] Gessi, S; Varani, K; Merighi, S; Cattabriga, E; Pancaldi, C; Szabadkai, Y; Rizzuto, R; Klotz, KN; Leung, E; Mac Lennan, S; Baraldi, PG; Borea, PA. Expression, pharmacological profile, and functional coupling of A2B receptors in a recombinant system and in peripheral blood cells using a novel selective antagonist radioligand, [3H]MRE 2029-F20. *Molecular pharmacology*, 2005, 67 (6), 2137-47.

[121] Lappas, CM; Rieger, JM; Linden, J. A2A adenosine receptor induction inhibits IFN-gamma production in murine CD4+ T cells. *Journal of immunology*, 2005, 174 (2), 1073-80.

[122] Takahashi, HK; Iwagaki, H; Hamano, R; Kanke, T; Liu, K; Sadamori, H; Yagi, T; Yoshino, T; Sendo, T; Tanaka, N; Nishibori, M. Effect of adenosine receptor subtypes stimulation on mixed lymphocyte reaction. *European journal of pharmacology*, 2007, 564 (1-3), 204-10.

[123] Raskovalova, T; Huang, X; Sitkovsky, M; Zacharia, LC; Jackson, EK; Gorelik, E. Gs protein-coupled adenosine receptor signaling and lytic function of activated NK cells. *Journal of immunology*, 2005, 175 (7), 4383-91.

[124] Raskovalova, T; Lokshin, A; Huang, X; Jackson, EK; Gorelik, E. Adenosine-mediated inhibition of cytotoxic activity and cytokine production by IL-2/NKp46-activated NK cells: involvement of protein kinase A isozyme I (PKA I). *Immunologic research*, 2006, 36 (1-3), 91-9.

[125] Priebe, T; Platsoucas, CD; Nelson, JA. Adenosine receptors and modulation of natural killer cell activity by purine nucleosides. *Cancer research*, 1990, 50 (14), 4328-31.

[126] Banchereau, J; Steinman, RM. Dendritic cells and the control of immunity. *Nature*, 1998, 392 (6673), 245-52.

[127] Macagno, A; Napolitani, G; Lanzavecchia, A; Sallusto, F. Duration, combination and timing: the signal integration model of dendritic cell activation. *Trends in immunology*, 2007, 28 (5), 227-33.

[128] Panther, E; Idzko, M; Herouy, Y; Rheinen, H; Gebicke-Haerter, PJ; Mrowietz, U; Dichmann, S; Norgauer, J. Expression and function of adenosine receptors in human dendritic cells. *FASEB journal: official publication of the Federation of American Societies for Experimental Biology*, 2001, 15 (11), 1963-70.

[129] Sexl, V; Mancusi, G; Holler, C; Gloria-Maercker, E; Schutz, W; Freissmuth, M. Stimulation of the mitogen-activated protein kinase via the A2A-adenosine receptor in primary human endothelial cells. *The Journal of biological chemistry*, 1997, 272 (9), 5792-9.

[130] Deguchi, H; Takeya, H; Urano, H; Gabazza, EC; Zhou, H; Suzuki, K. Adenosine regulates tissue factor expression on endothelial cells. *Thrombosis research*, 1998, 91 (2), 57-64.

[131] Olanrewaju, HA; Qin, W; Feoktistov, I; Scemama, JL; Mustafa, SJ. Adenosine A(2A) and A(2B) receptors in cultured human and porcine coronary artery endothelial cells. *American journal of physiology. Heart and circulatory physiology*, 2000, 279 (2), H650-6.

[132] Feoktistov, I; Goldstein, AE; Ryzhov, S; Zeng, D; Belardinelli, L; Voyno-Yasenetskaya, T; Biaggioni, I. Differential expression of adenosine receptors in human

endothelial cells: role of A2B receptors in angiogenic factor regulation. *Circulation research*, 2002, 90 (5), 531-8.

[133] Feoktistov, I; Ryzhov, S; Zhong, H; Goldstein, AE; Matafonov, A; Zeng, D; Biaggioni, I. Hypoxia modulates adenosine receptors in human endothelial and smooth muscle cells toward an A2B angiogenic phenotype. *Hypertension*, 2004, 44 (5), 649-54.

[134] Zernecke, A; Bidzhekov, K; Ozuyaman, B; Fraemohs, L; Liehn, EA; Luscher-Firzlaff, JM; Luscher, B; Schrader, J; Weber, C. CD73/ecto-5'-nucleotidase protects against vascular inflammation and neointima formation. *Circulation*, 2006, 113 (17), 2120-7.

[135] Wilson, CN; Batra, VK. Lipopolysaccharide binds to and activates A(1) adenosine receptors on human pulmonary artery endothelial cells. *Journal of endotoxin research*, 2002, 8 (4), 263-71.

[136] Cronstein, BN; Levin, RI; Philips, M; Hirschhorn, R; Abramson, SB; Weissmann, G. Neutrophil adherence to endothelium is enhanced via adenosine A1 receptors and inhibited via adenosine A2 receptors. *Journal of immunology*, 1992, 148 (7), 2201-6.

[137] Neely, CF; Keith, IM. A1 adenosine receptor antagonists block ischemia-reperfusion injury of the lung. *The American journal of physiology*, 1995, 268 (6 Pt 1), L1036-46.

[138] Neely, CF; DiPierro, FV; Kong, M; Greelish, JP; Gardner, TJ. A1 adenosine receptor antagonists block ischemia-reperfusion injury of the heart. *Circulation*, 1996, 94 (9 Suppl), II376-80.

[139] Forman, MB; Vitola, JV; Velasco, CE; Murray, JJ; Dubey, RK; Jackson, EK. Sustained reduction in myocardial reperfusion injury with an adenosine receptor antagonist: possible role of the neutrophil chemoattractant response. *The Journal of pharmacology and experimental therapeutics*, 2000, 292 (3), 929-38.

[140] Auchampach, JA; Jin, X; Moore, J; Wan, TC; Kreckler, LM; Ge, ZD; Narayanan, J; Whalley, E; Kiesman, W; Ticho, B; Smits, G; Gross, GJ. Comparison of three different A1 adenosine receptor antagonists on infarct size and multiple cycle ischemic preconditioning in anesthetized dogs. *The Journal of pharmacology and experimental therapeutics*, 2004, 308 (3), 846-56.

[141] Net, M; Valero, R; Almenara, R; Barros, P; Capdevila, L; Lopez-Boado, MA; Ruiz, A; Sanchez-Crivaro, F; Miquel, R; Deulofeu, R; Taura, P; Manyalich, M; Garcia-Valdecasas, JC. The effect of normothermic recirculation is mediated by ischemic preconditioning in NHBD liver transplantation. *American journal of transplantation : official journal of the American Society of Transplantation and the American Society of Transplant Surgeons*, 2005, 5 (10), 2385-92.

[142] Magata, S; Taniguchi, M; Suzuki, T; Shimamura, T; Fukai, M; Furukawa, H; Fujita, M; Todo, S. The effect of antagonism of adenosine A1 receptor against ischemia and reperfusion injury of the liver. *The Journal of surgical research*, 2007, 139 (1), 7-14.

[143] Satoh, A; Shimosegawa, T; Satoh, K; Ito, H; Kohno, Y; Masamune, A; Fujita, M; Toyota, T. Activation of adenosine A1-receptor pathway induces edema formation in the pancreas of rats. *Gastroenterology*, 2000, 119 (3), 829-36.

[144] Nadeem, A; Obiefuna, PC; Wilson, CN; Mustafa, SJ. Adenosine A1 receptor antagonist versus montelukast on airway reactivity and inflammation. *European journal of pharmacology*, 2006, 551 (1-3), 116-24.

[145] Ponnoth, DS; Nadeem, A; Mustafa, SJ. Adenosine-mediated alteration of vascular reactivity and inflammation in a murine model of asthma. *American journal of physiology. Heart and circulatory physiology*, 2008, 294 (5), H2158-65.

[146] Lee, DL; Bell, TD; Bhupatkar, J; Solis, G; Welch, WJ. Adenosine A1-receptor knockout mice have a decreased blood pressure response to low-dose ANG II infusion. *American journal of physiology. Regulatory, integrative and comparative physiology*, 2012, 303 (6), R683-8.

[147] Joo, JD; Kim, M; Horst, P; Kim, J; D'Agati, VD; Emala, CW. Sr; Lee, HT. Acute and delayed renal protection against renal ischemia and reperfusion injury with A1 adenosine receptors. *American journal of physiology. Renal physiology*, 2007, 293 (6), F1847-57.

[148] Lee, HT; Kim, M; Jan, M; Penn, RB; Emala, CW. Renal tubule necrosis and apoptosis modulation by A1 adenosine receptor expression. *Kidney international*, 2007, 71 (12), 1249-61.

[149] Hasko, G; Pacher, P. A2A receptors in inflammation and injury: lessons learned from transgenic animals. *Journal of leukocyte biology*, 2008, 83 (3), 447-55.

[150] Pinhal-Enfield, G; Ramanathan, M; Hasko, G; Vogel, SN; Salzman, AL; Boons, GJ; Leibovich, SJ. An angiogenic switch in macrophages involving synergy between Toll-like receptors 2, 4, 7, and 9 and adenosine A(2A) receptors. *The American journal of pathology*, 2003, 163 (2), 711-21.

[151] Panther, E; Corinti, S; Idzko, M; Herouy, Y; Napp, M; la Sala, A; Girolomoni, G; Norgauer, J. Adenosine affects expression of membrane molecules, cytokine and chemokine release, and the T-cell stimulatory capacity of human dendritic cells. *Blood*, 2003, 101 (10), 3985-90.

[152] Montesinos, MC; Desai, A; Chen, JF; Yee, H; Schwarzschild, MA; Fink, JS; Cronstein, BN. Adenosine promotes wound healing and mediates angiogenesis in response to tissue injury via occupancy of A(2A) receptors. *The American journal of pathology*, 2002, 160 (6), 2009-18.

[153] Naganuma, M; Wiznerowicz, EB; Lappas, CM; Linden, J; Worthington, MT; Ernst, PB. Cutting edge: Critical role for A2A adenosine receptors in the T cell-mediated regulation of colitis. *Journal of immunology*, 2006, 177 (5), 2765-9.

[154] Day, YJ; Marshall, MA; Huang, L; McDuffie, MJ; Okusa, MD; Linden, J. Protection from ischemic liver injury by activation of A2A adenosine receptors during reperfusion: inhibition of chemokine induction. *American journal of physiology. Gastrointestinal and liver physiology*, 2004, 286 (2), G285-93.

[155] Day, YJ; Huang, L; McDuffie, MJ; Rosin, DL; Ye, H; Chen, JF; Schwarzschild, MA; Fink, JS; Linden, J; Okusa, MD. Renal protection from ischemia mediated by A2A adenosine receptors on bone marrow-derived cells. *The Journal of clinical investigation*, 2003, 112 (6), 883-91.

[156] Lasley, RD; Jahania, MS; Mentzer, RM, Jr. Beneficial effects of adenosine A(2a) agonist CGS-21680 in infarcted and stunned porcine myocardium. *American journal of physiology. Heart and circulatory physiology*, 2001, 280 (4), H1660-6.

[157] Glover, DK; Riou, LM; Ruiz, M; Sullivan, GW; Linden, J; Rieger, JM; Macdonald, TL; Watson, DD; Beller, GA. Reduction of infarct size and postischemic inflammation from ATL-146e, a highly selective adenosine A2A receptor agonist, in reperfused canine myocardium. *American journal of physiology. Heart and circulatory physiology*, 2005, 288 (4), H1851-8.

[158] Ross, SD; Tribble, CG; Linden, J; Gangemi, JJ; Lanpher, BC; Wang, AY; Kron, IL. Selective adenosine-A2A activation reduces lung reperfusion injury following

transplantation. *The Journal of heart and lung transplantation: the official publication of the International Society for Heart Transplantation*, 1999, 18 (10), 994-1002.

[159] Reece, TB; Okonkwo, DO; Ellman, PI; Warren, PS; Smith, RL; Hawkins, AS; Linden, J; Kron, IL; Tribble, CG; Kern, JA. The evolution of ischemic spinal cord injury in function, cytoarchitecture, and inflammation and the effects of adenosine A2A receptor activation. *The Journal of thoracic and cardiovascular surgery*, 2004, 128 (6), 925-32.

[160] Luijk, B; van den Berge, M; Kerstjens, HA; Postma, DS; Cass, L; Sabin, A; Lammers, JW. Effect of an inhaled adenosine A2A agonist on the allergen-induced late asthmatic response. *Allergy*, 2008, 63 (1), 75-80.

[161] Mohsenin, A; Mi, T; Xia, Y; Kellems, RE; Chen, JF; Blackburn, MR. Genetic removal of the A2A adenosine receptor enhances pulmonary inflammation, mucin production, and angiogenesis in adenosine deaminase-deficient mice. *American journal of physiology. Lung cellular and molecular physiology*, 2007, 293 (3), L753-61.

[162] Ohta, A; Gorelik, E; Prasad, SJ; Ronchese, F; Lukashev, D; Wong, MK; Huang, X; Caldwell, S; Liu, K; Smith, P; Chen, JF; Jackson, EK; Apasov, S; Abrams, S; Sitkovsky, M. A2A adenosine receptor protects tumors from antitumor T cells. *Proceedings of the National Academy of Sciences of the United States of America*, 2006, 103 (35), 13132-7.

[163] Xaus, J; Mirabet, M; Lloberas, J; Soler, C; Lluis, C; Franco, R; Celada, A. IFN-gamma up-regulates the A2B adenosine receptor expression in macrophages: a mechanism of macrophage deactivation. *Journal of immunology*, 1999, 162 (6), 3607-14.

[164] Eltzschig, HK; Ibla, JC; Furuta, GT; Leonard, MO; Jacobson, KA; Enjyoji, K; Robson, SC; Colgan, SP. Coordinated adenine nucleotide phosphohydrolysis and nucleoside signaling in posthypoxic endothelium: role of ectonucleotidases and adenosine A2B receptors. *The Journal of experimental medicine*, 2003, 198 (5), 783-96.

[165] Ritchie, PK; Spangelo, BL; Krzymowski, DK; Rossiter, TB; Kurth, E; Judd, AM. Adenosine increases interleukin 6 release and decreases tumour necrosis factor release from rat adrenal zona glomerulosa cells, ovarian cells, anterior pituitary cells, and peritoneal macrophages. *Cytokine*, 1997, 9 (3), 187-98.

[166] Zhong, H; Wu, Y; Belardinelli, L; Zeng, D. A2B adenosine receptors induce IL-19 from bronchial epithelial cells, resulting in TNF-alpha increase. *American journal of respiratory cell and molecular biology*, 2006, 35 (5), 587-92.

[167] Feoktistov, I; Goldstein, AE; Biaggioni, I. Role of p38 mitogen-activated protein kinase and extracellular signal-regulated protein kinase kinase in adenosine A2B receptor-mediated interleukin-8 production in human mast cells. *Molecular pharmacology*, 1999, 55 (4), 726-34.

[168] Sitaraman, SV; Merlin, D; Wang, L; Wong, M; Gewirtz, AT; Si-Tahar, M; Madara, JL. Neutrophil-epithelial crosstalk at the intestinal lumenal surface mediated by reciprocal secretion of adenosine and IL-6. *The Journal of clinical investigation*, 2001, 107 (7), 861-9.

[169] Sajjadi, FG; Takabayashi, K; Foster, AC; Domingo, RC; Firestein, GS. Inhibition of TNF-alpha expression by adenosine: role of A3 adenosine receptors. *Journal of immunology*, 1996, 156 (9), 3435-42.

[170] Martin, L; Pingle, SC; Hallam, DM; Rybak, LP; Ramkumar, V. Activation of the adenosine A3 receptor in RAW 264.7 cells inhibits lipopolysaccharide-stimulated tumor necrosis factor-alpha release by reducing calcium-dependent activation of

nuclear factor-kappaB and extracellular signal-regulated kinase 1/2. *The Journal of pharmacology and experimental therapeutics*, 2006, 316 (1), 71-8.

[171] Chen, Y; Corriden, R; Inoue, Y; Yip, L; Hashiguchi, N; Zinkernagel, A; Nizet, V; Insel, PA; Junger, WG. ATP release guides neutrophil chemotaxis via P2Y2 and A3 receptors. *Science*, 2006, 314 (5806), 1792-5.

[172] Auchampach, JA; Jin, X; Wan, TC; Caughey, GH; Linden, J. Canine mast cell adenosine receptors: cloning and expression of the A3 receptor and evidence that degranulation is mediated by the A2B receptor. *Molecular pharmacology*, 1997, 52 (5), 846-60.

[173] Gao, Z; Li, BS; Day, YJ; Linden, J. A3 adenosine receptor activation triggers phosphorylation of protein kinase B and protects rat basophilic leukemia 2H3 mast cells from apoptosis. *Molecular pharmacology*, 2001, 59 (1), 76-82.

[174] Young, HW; Molina, JG; Dimina, D; Zhong, H; Jacobson, M; Chan, LN; Chan, TS; Lee, JJ; Blackburn, MR. A3 adenosine receptor signaling contributes to airway inflammation and mucus production in adenosine deaminase-deficient mice. *Journal of immunology*, 2004, 173 (2), 1380-9.

[175] Ezeamuzie, CI. Involvement of A(3) receptors in the potentiation by adenosine of the inhibitory effect of theophylline on human eosinophil degranulation: possible novel mechanism of the anti-inflammatory action of theophylline. *Biochemical pharmacology*, 2001, 61 (12), 1551-9.

[176] Morschl, E; Molina, JG; Volmer, JB; Mohsenin, A; Pero, RS; Hong, JS; Kheradmand, F; Lee, JJ; Blackburn, MR. A3 adenosine receptor signaling influences pulmonary inflammation and fibrosis. *American journal of respiratory cell and molecular biology*, 2008, 39 (6), 697-705.

[177] Ren, T; Qiu, Y; Wu, W; Feng, X; Ye, S; Wang, Z; Tian, T; He, Y; Yu, C; Zhou, Y. Activation of adenosine A3 receptor alleviates TNF-alpha-induced inflammation through inhibition of the NF-kappaB signaling pathway in human colonic epithelial cells. *Mediators of inflammation*, 2014, 2014, 818251.

[178] Matot, I; Weiniger, CF; Zeira, E; Galun, E; Joshi, BV; Jacobson, KA. A3 adenosine receptors and mitogen-activated protein kinases in lung injury following in vivo reperfusion. *Critical care*, 2006, 10 (2), R65.

[179] Fishman, P; Bar-Yehuda, S; Madi, L; Rath-Wolfson, L; Ochaion, A; Cohen, S; Baharav, E. The PI3K-NF-kappaB signal transduction pathway is involved in mediating the anti-inflammatory effect of IB-MECA in adjuvant-induced arthritis. *Arthritis research & therapy*, 2006, 8 (1), R33.

[180] Ochaion, A; Bar-Yehuda, S; Cohen, S; Amital, H; Jacobson, KA; Joshi, BV; Gao, ZG; Barer, F; Patoka, R; Del Valle, L; Perez-Liz, G; Fishman, P. The A3 adenosine receptor agonist CF502 inhibits the PI3K, PKB/Akt and NF-kappaB signaling pathway in synoviocytes from rheumatoid arthritis patients and in adjuvant-induced arthritis rats. *Biochemical pharmacology*, 2008, 76 (4), 482-94.

[181] Bar-Yehuda, S; Luger, D; Ochaion, A; Cohen, S; Patokaa, R; Zozulya, G; Silver, PB; de Morales, JM; Caspi, RR; Fishman, P. Inhibition of experimental auto-immune uveitis by the A3 adenosine receptor agonist CF101. *International journal of molecular medicine*, 2011, 28 (5), 727-31.

[182] Rosenberg, HF; Phipps, S; Foster, PS. Eosinophil trafficking in allergy and asthma. *The Journal of allergy and clinical immunology*, 2007, 119 (6), 1303-10; quiz 1311-2.

[183] Hammad, H; Lambrecht, BN. Lung dendritic cell migration. *Advances in immunology*, 2007, 93, 265-78.

[184] Kallinich, T; Beier, KC; Wahn, U; Stock, P; Hamelmann, E. T-cell co-stimulatory molecules: their role in allergic immune reactions. *The European respiratory journal*, 2007, 29 (6), 1246-55.

[185] Beier, KC; Kallinich, T; Hamelmann, E. T-cell co-stimulatory molecules: novel targets for the treatment of allergic airway disease. *The European respiratory journal*, 2007, 30 (2), 383-90.

[186] Lloyd, CM; Robinson, DS. Allergen-induced airway remodelling. *The European respiratory journal*, 2007, 29 (5), 1020-32.

[187] Holgate, ST. The epithelium takes centre stage in asthma and atopic dermatitis. *Trends in immunology*, 2007, 28 (6), 248-51.

[188] Gil, FR; Lauzon, AM. Smooth muscle molecular mechanics in airway hyperresponsiveness and asthma. *Canadian journal of physiology and pharmacology*, 2007, 85 (1), 133-40.

[189] An, SS; Bai, TR; Bates, JH; Black, JL; Brown, RH; Brusasco, V; Chitano, P; Deng, L; Dowell, M; Eidelman, DH; Fabry, B; Fairbank, NJ; Ford, LE; Fredberg, JJ; Gerthoffer, WT; Gilbert, SH; Gosens, R; Gunst, SJ; Halayko, AJ; Ingram, RH; Irvin, CG; James, AL; Janssen, LJ; King, GG; Knight, DA; Lauzon, AM; Lakser, OJ; Ludwig, MS; Lutchen, KR; Maksym, GN; Martin, JG; Mauad, T; McParland, BE; Mijailovich, SM; Mitchell, HW; Mitchell, RW; Mitzner, W; Murphy, TM; Pare, PD; Pellegrino, R; Sanderson, MJ; Schellenberg, RR; Seow, CY; Silveira, PS; Smith, PG; Solway, J; Stephens, NL; Sterk, PJ; Stewart, AG; Tang, DD; Tepper, RS; Tran, T; Wang, L. Airway smooth muscle dynamics: a common pathway of airway obstruction in asthma. *The European respiratory journal*, 2007, 29 (5), 834-60.

[190] Bucchioni, E; Csoma, Z; Allegra, L; Chung, KF; Barnes, PJ; Kharitonov, SA. Adenosine 5'-monophosphate increases levels of leukotrienes in breath condensate in asthma. *Respiratory medicine*, 2004, 98 (7), 651-5.

[191] Csoma, Z; Huszar, E; Vizi, E; Vass, G; Szabo, Z; Herjavecz, I; Kollai, M; Horvath, I. Adenosine level in exhaled breath increases during exercise-induced bronchoconstriction. *The European respiratory journal*, 2005, 25 (5), 873-8.

[192] Polosa, R. Adenosine-receptor subtypes: their relevance to adenosine-mediated responses in asthma and chronic obstructive pulmonary disease. *The European respiratory journal*, 2002, 20 (2), 488-96.

[193] Livingston, M; Heaney, LG; Ennis, M. Adenosine, inflammation and asthma--a review. *Inflammation research: official journal of the European Histamine Research Society ... [et al.]*, 2004, 53 (5), 171-8.

[194] Keir, S; Boswell-Smith, V; Spina, D; Page, C. Mechanism of adenosine-induced airways obstruction in allergic guinea pigs. *British journal of pharmacology*, 2006, 147 (7), 720-8.

[195] Hua, X; Erikson, CJ; Chason, KD; Rosebrock, CN; Deshpande, DA; Penn, RB; Tilley, SL. Involvement of A1 adenosine receptors and neural pathways in adenosine-induced bronchoconstriction in mice. *American journal of physiology. Lung cellular and molecular physiology*, 2007, 293 (1), L25-32.

[196] Bochenek, G; Nizankowska, E; Gielicz, A; Szczeklik, A. Mast cell activation after adenosine inhalation challenge in patients with bronchial asthma. *Allergy*, 2008, 63 (1), 140-1.

[197] Vestbo, J; Hurd, SS; Agusti, AG; Jones, PW; Vogelmeier, C; Anzueto, A; Barnes, PJ; Fabbri, LM; Martinez, FJ; Nishimura, M; Stockley, RA; Sin, DD; Rodriguez-Roisin, R. Global strategy for the diagnosis, management, and prevention of chronic obstructive pulmonary disease: GOLD executive summary. *American journal of respiratory and critical care medicine*, 2013, 187 (4), 347-65.

[198] Fan, M; Qin, W; Mustafa, SJ. Characterization of adenosine receptor(s) involved in adenosine-induced bronchoconstriction in an allergic mouse model. *American journal of physiology. Lung cellular and molecular physiology*, 2003, 284 (6), L1012-9.

[199] Press, NJ; Taylor, RJ; Fullerton, JD; Tranter, P; McCarthy, C; Keller, TH; Brown, L; Cheung, R; Christie, J; Haberthuer, S; Hatto, JD; Keenan, M; Mercer, MK; Press, NE; Sahri, H; Tuffnell, AR; Tweed, M; Fozard, JR. A new orally bioavailable dual adenosine A2B/A3 receptor antagonist with therapeutic potential. *Bioorganic & medicinal chemistry letters*, 2005, 15 (12), 3081-5.

[200] Rivo, J; Zeira, E; Galun, E; Matot, I. Activation of A3 adenosine receptor provides lung protection against ischemia-reperfusion injury associated with reduction in apoptosis. *American journal of transplantation:official journal of the American Society of Transplantation and the American Society of Transplant Surgeons*, 2004, 4 (12), 1941-8.

[201] Rivo, J; Zeira, E; Galun, E; Matot, I. Activation of A3 adenosine receptors attenuates lung injury after in vivo reperfusion. *Anesthesiology*, 2004, 101 (5), 1153-9.

[202] Lee, HT; Gallos, G; Nasr, SH; Emala, CW. A1 adenosine receptor activation inhibits inflammation, necrosis, and apoptosis after renal ischemia-reperfusion injury in mice. *Journal of the American Society of Nephrology : JASN*, 2004, 15 (1), 102-11.

[203] Lee, HT; Ota-Setlik, A; Xu, H; D'Agati, VD; Jacobson, MA; Emala, CW. A3 adenosine receptor knockout mice are protected against ischemia- and myoglobinuria-induced renal failure. *American journal of physiology. Renal physiology*, 2003, 284 (2), F267-73.

[204] Lee, HT; Emala, CW. Protective effects of renal ischemic preconditioning and adenosine pretreatment: role of A(1) and A(3) receptors. *American journal of physiology. Renal physiology*, 2000, 278 (3), F380-7.

[205] Yang, H; Avila, MY; Peterson-Yantorno, K; Coca-Prados, M; Stone, RA; Jacobson, KA; Civan, MM. The cross-species A3 adenosine-receptor antagonist MRS 1292 inhibits adenosine-triggered human nonpigmented ciliary epithelial cell fluid release and reduces mouse intraocular pressure. *Current eye research*, 2005, 30 (9), 747-54.

[206] Wang, Z; Do, CW; Avila, MY; Peterson-Yantorno, K; Stone, RA; Gao, ZG; Joshi, B; Besada, P; Jeong, LS; Jacobson, KA; Civan, MM. Nucleoside-derived antagonists to A3 adenosine receptors lower mouse intraocular pressure and act across species. *Experimental eye research*, 2010, 90 (1), 146-54.

[207] Taylor, CT; Colgan, SP. Hypoxia and gastrointestinal disease. *Journal of molecular medicine*, 2007, 85 (12), 1295-300.

[208] Sundaram, U; Hassanain, H; Suntres, Z; Yu, JG; Cooke, HJ; Guzman, J; Christofi, FL. Rabbit chronic ileitis leads to up-regulation of adenosine A1/A3 gene products,

oxidative stress, and immune modulation. *Biochemical pharmacology*, 2003, 65 (9), 1529-38.

[209] Kolachala, V; Asamoah, V; Wang, L; Obertone, TS; Ziegler, TR; Merlin, D; Sitaraman, SV. TNF-alpha upregulates adenosine 2b (A2b) receptor expression and signaling in intestinal epithelial cells: a basis for A2bR overexpression in colitis. *Cellular and molecular life sciences : CMLS*, 2005, 62 (22), 2647-57.

[210] Lee, HT; Kim, M; Joo, JD; Gallos, G; Chen, JF; Emala, CW. A3 adenosine receptor activation decreases mortality and renal and hepatic injury in murine septic peritonitis. *American journal of physiology. Regulatory, integrative and comparative physiology*, 2006, 291 (4), R959-69.

[211] Mabley, J; Soriano, F; Pacher, P; Hasko, G; Marton, A; Wallace, R; Salzman, A; Szabo, C. The adenosine A3 receptor agonist, N6-(3-iodobenzyl)-adenosine-5'-N-methyluronamide, is protective in two murine models of colitis. *European journal of pharmacology*, 2003, 466 (3), 323-9.

[212] Ren, T; Tian, T; Feng, X; Ye, S; Wang, H; Wu, W; Qiu, Y; Yu, C; He, Y; Zeng, J; Cen, J; Zhou, Y. An adenosine A3 receptor agonist inhibits DSS-induced colitis in mice through modulation of the NF-kappaB signaling pathway. *Scientific reports*, 2015, 5, 9047.

[213] Baharav, E; Bar-Yehuda, S; Madi, L; Silberman, D; Rath-Wolfson, L; Halpren, M; Ochaion, A; Weinberger, A; Fishman, P. Antiinflammatory effect of A3 adenosine receptor agonists in murine autoimmune arthritis models. *The Journal of rheumatology*, 2005, 32 (3), 469-76.

[214] Rath-Wolfson, L; Bar-Yehuda, S; Madi, L; Ochaion, A; Cohen, S; Zabutti, A; Fishman, P. IB-MECA, an A3 adenosine receptor agonist prevents bone resorption in rats with adjuvant induced arthritis. *Clinical and experimental rheumatology*, 2006, 24 (4), 400-6.

[215] Ochaion, A; Bar-Yehuda, S; Cohn, S; Del Valle, L; Perez-Liz, G; Madi, L; Barer, F; Farbstein, M; Fishman-Furman, S; Reitblat, T; Reitblat, A; Amital, H; Levi, Y; Molad, Y; Mader, R; Tishler, M; Langevitz, P; Zabutti, A; Fishman, P. Methotrexate enhances the anti-inflammatory effect of CF101 via up-regulation of the A3 adenosine receptor expression. *Arthritis research & therapy*, 2006, 8 (6), R169.

[216] Chan, ES; Cronstein, BN. Molecular action of methotrexate in inflammatory diseases. *Arthritis research*, 2002, 4 (4), 266-73.

[217] Laghi Pasini, F; Capecchi, PL; Di Perri, T. Adenosine plasma levels after low dose methotrexate administration. *The Journal of rheumatology*, 1997, 24 (12), 2492-3.

[218] Baggott, JE; Morgan, SL; Sams, WM; Linden, J. Urinary adenosine and aminoimidazolecarboxamide excretion in methotrexate-treated patients with psoriasis. *Archives of dermatology*, 1999, 135 (7), 813-7.

[219] Silverman, MH; Strand, V; Markovits, D; Nahir, M; Reitblat, T; Molad, Y; Rosner, I; Rozenbaum, M; Mader, R; Adawi, M; Caspi, D; Tishler, M; Langevitz, P; Rubinow, A; Friedman, J; Green, L; Tanay, A; Ochaion, A; Cohen, S; Kerns, WD; Cohn, I; Fishman-Furman, S; Farbstein, M; Yehuda, SB; Fishman, P. Clinical evidence for utilization of the A3 adenosine receptor as a target to treat rheumatoid arthritis: data from a phase II clinical trial. *The Journal of rheumatology*, 2008, 35 (1), 41-8.

[220] Guzman-Aranguez, A; Gasull, X; Diebold, Y; Pintor, J. Purinergic receptors in ocular inflammation. *Mediators of inflammation*, 2014, 2014, 320906.

[221] Boehm, N; Riechardt, AI; Wiegand, M; Pfeiffer, N; Grus, FH. Proinflammatory cytokine profiling of tears from dry eye patients by means of antibody microarrays. *Investigative ophthalmology & visual science*, 2011, 52 (10), 7725-30.

[222] Lam, H; Bleiden, L; de Paiva, CS; Farley, W; Stern, ME; Pflugfelder, SC. Tear cytokine profiles in dysfunctional tear syndrome. *American journal of ophthalmology*, 2009, 147 (2), 198-205 e1.

[223] Stevenson, W; Chauhan, SK; Dana, R. Dry eye disease: an immune-mediated ocular surface disorder. *Archives of ophthalmology*, 2012, 130 (1), 90-100.

[224] Avni, I; Garzozi, HJ; Barequet, IS; Segev, F; Varssano, D; Sartani, G; Chetrit, N; Bakshi, E; Zadok, D; Tomkins, O; Litvin, G; Jacobson, KA; Fishman, S; Harpaz, Z; Farbstein, M; Yehuda, SB; Silverman, MH; Kerns, WD; Bristol, DR; Cohn, I; Fishman, P. Treatment of dry eye syndrome with orally administered CF101: data from a phase 2 clinical trial. *Ophthalmology*, 2010, 117 (7), 1287-93.

[225] Menter, A; Korman, NJ; Elmets, CA; Feldman, SR; Gelfand, JM; Gordon, KB; Gottlieb, A; Koo, JY; Lebwohl, M; Lim, HW; Van Voorhees, AS; Beutner, KR; Bhushan, R. Guidelines of care for the management of psoriasis and psoriatic arthritis: Section 5. Guidelines of care for the treatment of psoriasis with phototherapy and photochemotherapy. *Journal of the American Academy of Dermatology*, 2010, 62 (1), 114-35.

[226] Kofoed, K; Skov, L; Zachariae, C. New drugs and treatment targets in psoriasis. *Acta dermato-venereologica*, 2015, 95 (2), 133-9.

[227] Gessi, S; Merighi, S; Borea, PA. Targeting adenosine receptors to prevent inflammatory skin diseases. *Experimental dermatology*, 2014, 23 (8), 553-4.

[228] Arasa, J; Martos, P; Terencio, MC; Valcuende-Cavero, F; Montesinos, MC. Topical application of the adenosine A2A receptor agonist CGS-21680 prevents phorbol-induced epidermal hyperplasia and inflammation in mice. *Experimental dermatology*, 2014, 23 (8), 555-60.

[229] Greenberg, B; Thomas, I; Banish, D; Goldman, S; Havranek, E; Massie, BM; Zhu, Y; Ticho, B; Abraham, WT. Effects of multiple oral doses of an A1 adenosine antagonist, BG9928, in patients with heart failure: results of a placebo-controlled, dose-escalation study. *Journal of the American College of Cardiology*, 2007, 50 (7), 600-6.

[230] Givertz, MM; Massie, BM; Fields, TK; Pearson, LL; Dittrich, HC; Cki; Investigators, C. KI. The effects of KW-3902, an adenosine A1-receptor antagonist, on diuresis and renal function in patients with acute decompensated heart failure and renal impairment or diuretic resistance. *Journal of the American College of Cardiology*, 2007, 50 (16), 1551-60.

[231] Dittrich, HC; Gupta, DK; Hack, TC; Dowling, T; Callahan, J; Thomson, S. The effect of KW-3902, an adenosine A1 receptor antagonist, on renal function and renal plasma flow in ambulatory patients with heart failure and renal impairment. *Journal of cardiac failure*, 2007, 13 (8), 609-17.

[232] Bar-Yehuda, S; Silverman, MH; Kerns, WD; Ochaion, A; Cohen, S; Fishman, P. The anti-inflammatory effect of A3 adenosine receptor agonists: a novel targeted therapy for rheumatoid arthritis. *Expert opinion on investigational drugs*, 2007, 16 (10), 1601-13.

[233] Fishman, P; Bar-Yehuda, S; Barer, F; Madi, L; Multani, AS; Pathak, S. The A3 adenosine receptor as a new target for cancer therapy and chemoprotection. *Exp Cell Res*, 2001, 269 (2), 230-6.

[234] Gerondakis, S; Fulford, TS; Messina, NL; Grumont, RJ. NF-kappaB control of T cell development. *Nat Immunol*, 2014, 15 (1), 15-25.

[235] Kim, GD; Oh, J; Jeong, LS; Lee, SK. Thio-Cl-IB-MECA, a novel A(3) adenosine receptor agonist, suppresses angiogenesis by regulating PI3K/AKT/mTOR and ERK signaling in endothelial cells. *Biochemical and Biophysical Research Communications*, 2013, 437 (1), 79-86.

[236] Kanno, T; Gotoh, A; Fujita, Y; Nakano, T; Nishizaki, T. A(3) adenosine receptor mediates apoptosis in 5637 human bladder cancer cells by G(q) protein/PKC-dependent AIF upregulation. *Cellular Physiology and Biochemistry*, 2012, 30 (5), 1159-68.

[237] Kim, TH; Kim, YK; Woo, JS. The adenosine A3 receptor agonist Cl-IB-MECA induces cell death through Ca(2)(+)/ROS-dependent down regulation of ERK and Akt in A172 human glioma cells. *Neurochem Res*, 2012, 37 (12), 2667-77.

[238] Kim, H; Kang, JW; Lee, S; Choi, WJ; Jeong, LS; Yang, Y; Hong, JT; DO YOUNG, Y. A3 adenosine receptor antagonist, truncated Thio-Cl-IB-MECA, induces apoptosis in T24 human bladder cancer cells. *Anticancer research*, 2010, 30 (7), 2823-2830.

[239] Barczyk, K; Ehrchen, J; Tenbrock, K; Ahlmann, M; Kneidl, J; Viemann, D; Roth, J. Glucocorticoids promote survival of anti-inflammatory macrophages via stimulation of adenosine receptor A3. *Blood*, 2010, 116 (3), 446-55.

[240] Merighi, S; Benini, A; Mirandola, P; Gessi, S; Varani, K; Leung, E; Maclennan, S; Baraldi, PG; Borea, PA. Modulation of the Akt/Ras/Raf/MEK/ERK pathway by A(3) adenosine receptor. *Purinergic Signal.*, 2006, 2 (4), 627-32.

[241] Duann, P; Ho, T.-Y; Desai, BD; Kapoian, T; Cowen, DS; Lianos, EA. Mesangial cell apoptosis induced by stimulation of the adenosine A3 receptor: signaling and apoptotic events. *Journal of investigative medicine*, 2005, 53 (1), 37-43.

[242] Hammarberg, C; Fredholm, BB; Schulte, G. Adenosine A3 receptor-mediated regulation of p38 and extracellular-regulated kinase ERK1/2 via phosphatidylinositol-3'-kinase. *Biochemical pharmacology*, 2004, 67 (1), 129-134.

[243] Graham, S; Combes, P; Crumiere, M; Klotz, K.-N; Dickenson, JM. Regulation of p42/p44 mitogen-activated protein kinase by the human adenosine A 3 receptor in transfected CHO cells. *European journal of pharmacology*, 2001, 420 (1), 19-26.

[244] Fishman, P; Madi, L; Bar-Yehuda, S; Barer, F; Del Valle, L; Khalili, K. Evidence for involvement of Wnt signaling pathway in IB-MECA mediated suppression of melanoma cells. *Oncogene*, 2002, 21 (25), 4060-4.

[245] Yoshikawa, N; Yamada, S; Takeuchi, C; Kagota, S; Shinozuka, K; Kunitomo, M; Nakamura, K. Cordycepin (3'-deoxyadenosine) inhibits the growth of B16-BL6 mouse melanoma cells through the stimulation of adenosine A3 receptor followed by glycogen synthase kinase-3beta activation and cyclin D1 suppression. *Naunyn-Schmiedebergs Archiv für Pharmakologie*, 2008, 377 (4-6), 591-5.

[246] Yang, J; Zheng, X; Haugen, F; Darè, E; Lövdahl, C; Schulte, G; Fredholm, B; Valen, G. Adenosine increases LPS-induced nuclear factor kappa B activation in smooth muscle cells via an intracellular mechanism and modulates it via actions on adenosine receptors. *Acta Physiologica*, 2014, 210 (3), 590-599.

[247] Morello, S; Sorrentino, R; Porta, A; Forte, G; Popolo, A; Petrella, A; Pinto, A. Cl-IB-MECA enhances TRAIL-induced apoptosis via the modulation of NF-kappaB signalling pathway in thyroid cancer cells. *J. Cell. Physiol.*, 2009, 221 (2), 378-86.

[248] Fishman, P; Bar-Yehuda, S; Ohana, G; Barer, F; Ochaion, A; Erlanger, A; Madi, L. An agonist to the A3 adenosine receptor inhibits colon carcinoma growth in mice via modulation of GSK-3 beta and NF-kappa B. *Oncogene*, 2004, 23 (14), 2465-71.

[249] Jajoo, S; Mukherjea, D; Watabe, K; Ramkumar, V. Adenosine A 3 receptor suppresses prostate cancer metastasis by inhibiting NADPH oxidase activity. *Neoplasia*, 2009, 11 (11), 1132-IN5.

[250] Abedi, H; Aghaei, M; Panjehpour, M; Hajiahmadi, S. Mitochondrial and caspase pathways are involved in the induction of apoptosis by IB-MECA in ovarian cancer cell lines. *Tumour. Biol.*, 2014, 35 (11), 11027-39.

[251] Aghaei, M; Panjehpour, M; Karami-Tehrani, F; Salami, S. Molecular mechanisms of A3 adenosine receptor-induced G1 cell cycle arrest and apoptosis in androgen-dependent and independent prostate cancer cell lines: involvement of intrinsic pathway. *Journal of Cancer Research and Clinical Oncology*, 2011, 137 (10), 1511-23.

[252] Otsuki, T-i; Kanno, T; Fujita, Y; Tabata, C; Fukuoka, K; Nakano, T; Gotoh, A; Nishizaki, T. A3 adenosine receptor-mediated p53-dependent apoptosis in Lu-65 human lung cancer cells. *Cellular Physiology and Biochemistry*, 2012, 30 (1), 210-220.

[253] Kanno, T; Gotoh, A; Fujita, Y; Nakano, T; Nishizaki, T. A3 adenosine receptor mediates apoptosis in 5637 human bladder cancer cells by Gq protein/PKC-dependent AIF upregulation. *Cellular Physiology and Biochemistry*, 2012, 30 (5), 1159-1168.

[254] Varani, K; Vincenzi, F; Targa, M; Paradiso, B; Parrilli, A; Fini, M; Lanza, G; Borea, PA. The stimulation of A(3) adenosine receptors reduces bone-residing breast cancer in a rat preclinical model. *Eur. J. Cancer.*, 2013, 49 (2), 482-91.

[255] Feoktistov, I; Ryzhov, S; Goldstein, AE; Biaggioni, I. Mast cell-mediated stimulation of angiogenesis: cooperative interaction between A2B and A3 adenosine receptors. *Circ. Res.*, 2003, 92 (5), 485-92.

[256] Merighi, S; Benini, A; Mirandola, P; Gessi, S; Varani, K; Leung, E; MacLennan, S; Baraldi, PG; Borea, PA. A3 Adenosine Receptors Modulate Hypoxia-inducible Factor-1a Expression in Human A375 Melanoma Cells. *Neoplasia*, 2005, 7 (10), 894-903.

[257] Hanahan, D; Weinberg, RA. The hallmarks of cancer. *Cell*, 2000, 100 (1), 57-70.

[258] Hinz, M; Krappmann, D; Eichten, A; Heder, A; Scheidereit, C; Strauss, M. NF-κB function in growth control: regulation of cyclin D1 expression and G0/G1-to-S-phase transition. *Mol. Cell. Biol.*, 1999, 19 (4), 2690-2698.

[259] Yang, K; Hitomi, M; Stacey, DW. Variations in cyclin D1 levels through the cell cycle determine the proliferative fate of a cell. *Cell Div.*, 2006, 1, 32.

[260] Miller, DM; Thomas, SD; Islam, A; Muench, D; Sedoris, K. c-Myc and cancer metabolism. *Clin. Cancer Res.*, 2012, 18 (20), 5546-53.

[261] Sheth, S; Brito, R; Mukherjea, D; Rybak, LP; Ramkumar, V. Adenosine receptors: expression, function and regulation. *Int. J. Mol. Sci.*, 2014, 15 (2), 2024-52.

[262] Synowitz, M; Glass, R; Farber, K; Markovic, D; Kronenberg, G; Herrmann, K; Schnermann, J; Nolte, C; van Rooijen, N; Kiwit, J; Kettenmann, H. A1 adenosine receptors in microglia control glioblastoma-host interaction. *Cancer Res.*, 2006, 66 (17), 8550-7.

[263] Beavis, PA; Divisekera, U; Paget, C; Chow, MT; John, LB; Devaud, C; Dwyer, K; Stagg, J; Smyth, MJ; Darcy, PK. Blockade of A2A receptors potently suppresses the metastasis of CD73+ tumors. *Proc. Natl. Acad. Sci. U. SA.*, 2013, 110 (36), 14711-6.

[264] Ahmad, A; Ahmad, S; Glover, L; Miller, SM; Shannon, JM; Guo, X; Franklin, WA; Bridges, JP; Schaack, JB; Colgan, SP; White, CW. Adenosine A2A receptor is a unique angiogenic target of HIF-2alpha in pulmonary endothelial cells. *Proc. Natl. Acad. Sci. U. SA.*, 2009, 106 (26), 10684-9.

[265] Ratcliffe, PJ. HIF-1 and HIF-2: working alone or together in hypoxia? *J. Clin. Invest.*, 2007, 117 (4), 862-5.

[266] Antonioli, L; Blandizzi, C; Pacher, P; Hasko, G. Immunity, inflammation and cancer: a leading role for adenosine. *Nat. Rev. Cancer*, 2013, 13 (12), 842-57.

[267] Fishman, P; Bar-Yehuda, S; Liang, BT; Jacobson, KA. Pharmacological and therapeutic effects of A3 adenosine receptor agonists. *Drug Discov Today*, 2012, 17 (7-8), 359-66.

[268] (a) Fishman, P; Madi, L; Bar-Yehuda, S; Barer, F; Del Valle, L; Khalili, K. Evidence for involvement of Wnt signaling pathway in IB-MECA mediated suppression of melanoma cells. *Oncogene*, 2002, 21 (25), 4060-4064. (b) Merighi, S; Benini, A; Mirandola, P; Gessi, S; Varani, K; Leung, E; Maclennan, S; Borea, PA. A3 adenosine receptor activation inhibits cell proliferation via phosphatidylinositol 3-kinase/Akt-dependent inhibition of the extracellular signal-regulated kinase 1/2 phosphorylation in A375 human melanoma cells. *J. Biol. Chem.*, 2005, 280 (20), 19516-26.

[269] Tsubaki, M; Matsuoka, H; Yamamoto, C; Kato, C; Ogaki, M; Satou, T; Itoh, T; Kusunoki, T; Tanimori, Y; Nishida, S. The protein kinase C inhibitor, H7, inhibits tumor cell invasion and metastasis in mouse melanoma via suppression of ERK1/2. *Clin. Exp. Metastasis*, 2007, 24 (6), 431-438.

[270] Jajoo, S; Mukherjea, D; Watabe, K; Ramkumar, V. Adenosine A(3) receptor suppresses prostate cancer metastasis by inhibiting NADPH oxidase activity. *Neoplasia*, 2009, 11 (11), 1132-45.

[271] Morello, S; Petrella, A; Festa, M; Popolo, A; Monaco, M; Vuttariello, E; Chiappetta, G; Parente, L; Pinto, A. Cl-IB-MECA inhibits human thyroid cancer cell proliferation independently of A3 adenosine receptor activation. *Cancer Biol. Ther.*, 2014, 7 (2), 278-284.

[272] Merighi, S; Varani, K; Gessi, S; Cattabriga, E; Iannotta, V; Ulouglu, C; Leung, E; Borea, PA. Pharmacological and biochemical characterization of adenosine receptors in the human malignant melanoma A375 cell line. *Br. J. Pharmacol.*, 2001, 134 (6), 1215-1226.

[273] Fredholm, BB; Irenius, E; Kull, B; Schulte, G. Comparison of the potency of adenosine as an agonist at human adenosine receptors expressed in Chinese hamster ovary cells. *Biochemical pharmacology*, 2001, 61 (4), 443-8.

[274] van Galen, PJ; van Bergen, AH; Gallo-Rodriguez, C; Melman, N; Olah, ME; AP, IJ; Stiles, GL; Jacobson, KA. A binding site model and structure-activity relationships for the rat A3 adenosine receptor. *Molecular pharmacology*, 1994, 45 (6), 1101-11.

[275] Gao, ZG; Blaustein, JB; Gross, AS; Melman, N; Jacobson, KA. N6-Substituted adenosine derivatives: selectivity, efficacy, and species differences at A3 adenosine receptors. *Biochemical pharmacology*, 2003, 65 (10), 1675-84.

[276] Gallo-Rodriguez, C; Ji, XD; Melman, N; Siegman, BD; Sanders, LH; Orlina, J; Fischer, B; Pu, Q; Olah, ME; van Galen, PJ; et al. Structure-activity relationships of N6-benzyladenosine-5'-uronamides as A3-selective adenosine agonists. *Journal of medicinal chemistry*, 1994, 37 (5), 636-46.

[277] Kim, HO; Ji, XD; Melman, N; Olah, ME; Stiles, GL; Jacobson, KA. Structure-activity relationships of 1,3-dialkylxanthine derivatives at rat A3 adenosine receptors. *Journal of medicinal chemistry*, 1994, 37 (20), 3373-82.

[278] Baraldi, PG; Cacciari, B; Spalluto, G; Ji, XD; Olah, ME; Stiles, G; Dionisotti, S; Zocchi, C; Ongini, E; Jacobson, KA. Novel N6-(substituted-phenylcarbamoyl)adenosine-5'-uronamides as potent agonists for A3 adenosine receptors. *Journal of medicinal chemistry*, 1996, 39 (3), 802-6.

[279] Klotz, KN; Camaioni, E; Volpini, R; Kachler, S; Vittori, S; Cristalli, G., 2-Substituted N-ethylcarboxamidoadenosine derivatives as high-affinity agonists at human A3 adenosine receptors. *Naunyn-Schmiedeberg's archives of pharmacology*, 1999, 360 (2), 103-8.

[280] Volpini, R; Costanzi, S; Lambertucci, C; Taffi, S; Vittori, S; Klotz, KN; Cristalli, G. N(6)-alkyl-2-alkynyl derivatives of adenosine as potent and selective agonists at the human adenosine A(3) receptor and a starting point for searching A(2B) ligands. *Journal of medicinal chemistry*, 2002, 45 (15), 3271-9.

[281] Klotz, KN; Falgner, N; Kachler, S; Lambertucci, C; Vittori, S; Volpini, R; Cristalli, G., [3H]HEMADO--a novel tritiated agonist selective for the human adenosine A3 receptor. *European journal of pharmacology*, 2007, 556 (1-3), 14-8.

[282] Cosyn, L; Palaniappan, KK; Kim, SK; Duong, HT; Gao, ZG; Jacobson, KA; Van Calenbergh, S., 2-triazole-substituted adenosines: a new class of selective A3 adenosine receptor agonists, partial agonists, and antagonists. *Journal of medicinal chemistry*, 2006, 49 (25), 7373-83.

[283] Zhu, R; Frazier, CR; Linden, J; Macdonald, TL. N6-ethyl-2-alkynyl NECAs, selective human A3 adenosine receptor agonists. *Bioorganic & medicinal chemistry letters*, 2006, 16 (9), 2416-8.

[284] Volpini, R; Dal Ben, D; Lambertucci, C; Taffi, S; Vittori, S; Klotz, KN; Cristalli, G. N6-methoxy-2-alkynyladenosine derivatives as highly potent and selective ligands at the human A3 adenosine receptor. *Journal of medicinal chemistry*, 2007, 50 (6), 1222-30.

[285] Ohno, M; Gao, ZG; Van Rompaey, P; Tchilibon, S; Kim, SK; Harris, BA; Gross, AS; Duong, HT; Van Calenbergh, S; Jacobson, KA. Modulation of adenosine receptor affinity and intrinsic efficacy in adenine nucleosides substituted at the 2-position. *Bioorganic & medicinal chemistry*, 2004, 12 (11), 2995-3007.

[286] Elzein, E; Palle, V; Wu, Y; Maa, T; Zeng, D; Zablocki, J. 2-Pyrazolyl-N(6)-substituted adenosine derivatives as high affinity and selective adenosine A(3) receptor agonists. *Journal of medicinal chemistry*, 2004, 47 (19), 4766-73.

[287] Kim, HO; Ji, XD; Siddiqi, SM; Olah, ME; Stiles, GL; Jacobson, KA. 2-Substitution of N6-benzyladenosine-5'-uronamides enhances selectivity for A3 adenosine receptors. *Journal of medicinal chemistry*, 1994, 37 (21), 3614-21.

[288] Mogensen, JP; Roberts, SM; Bowler, AN; Thomsen, C; Knutsen, LJ. The synthesis of new adenosine A3 selective ligands containing bioisosteric isoxazoles. *Bioorganic & medicinal chemistry letters*, 1998, 8 (13), 1767-70.

[289] DeNinno, MP; Masamune, H; Chenard, LK; DiRico, KJ; Eller, C; Etienne, JB; Tickner, JE; Kennedy, SP; Knight, DR; Kong, J; Oleynek, JJ; Tracey, WR; Hill, RJ. 3'-Aminoadenosine-5'-uronamides: discovery of the first highly selective agonist at the human adenosine A3 receptor. *Journal of medicinal chemistry*, 2003, 46 (3), 353-5.

[290] Jeong, LS; Jin, DZ; Kim, HO; Shin, DH; Moon, HR; Gunaga, P; Chun, MW; Kim, YC; Melman, N; Gao, ZG; Jacobson, KA. N6-substituted D-4'-thioadenosine-5'-methyluronamides: potent and selective agonists at the human A3 adenosine receptor. *Journal of medicinal chemistry*, 2003, 46 (18), 3775-7.

[291] Jeong, LS; Lee, HW; Jacobson, KA; Kim, HO; Shin, DH; Lee, JA; Gao, ZG; Lu, C; Duong, HT; Gunaga, P; Lee, SK; Jin, DZ; Chun, MW; Moon, HR. Structure-activity relationships of 2-chloro-N6-substituted-4'-thioadenosine-5'-uronamides as highly potent and selective agonists at the human A3 adenosine receptor. *Journal of medicinal chemistry*, 2006, 49 (1), 273-81.

[292] Jeong, LS; Lee, HW; Kim, HO; Tosh, DK; Pal, S; Choi, WJ; Gao, ZG; Patel, AR; Williams, W; Jacobson, KA; Kim, HD. Structure-activity relationships of 2-chloro-N6-substituted-4'-thioadenosine-5'-N,N-dialkyluronamides as human A3 adenosine receptor antagonists. *Bioorganic & medicinal chemistry letters*, 2008, 18 (5), 1612-6.

[293] Gao, ZG; Jeong, LS; Moon, HR; Kim, HO; Choi, WJ; Shin, DH; Elhalem, E; Comin, MJ; Melman, N; Mamedova, L; Gross, AS; Rodriguez, JB; Jacobson, KA. Structural determinants of efficacy at A3 adenosine receptors: modification of the ribose moiety. *Biochemical pharmacology*, 2004, 67 (5), 893-901.

[294] Jacobson, KA; Ji, X; Li, AH; Melman, N; Siddiqui, MA; Shin, KJ; Marquez, VE; Ravi, RG. Methanocarba analogues of purine nucleosides as potent and selective adenosine receptor agonists. *Journal of medicinal chemistry*, 2000, 43 (11), 2196-203.

[295] Ravi, G; Lee, K; Ji, X; Kim, HS; Soltysiak, KA; Marquez, VE; Jacobson, KA. Synthesis and purine receptor affinity of 6-oxopurine nucleosides and nucleotides containing (N)-methanocarba-pseudoribose rings. *Bioorganic & medicinal chemistry letters*, 2001, 11 (17), 2295-300.

[296] Gao, ZG; Kim, SK; Biadatti, T; Chen, W; Lee, K; Barak, D; Kim, SG; Johnson, CR; Jacobson, KA. Structural determinants of A(3) adenosine receptor activation: nucleoside ligands at the agonist/antagonist boundary. *Journal of medicinal chemistry*, 2002, 45 (20), 4471-84.

[297] Tchilibon, S; Joshi, BV; Kim, SK; Duong, HT; Gao, ZG; Jacobson, KA. (N)-methanocarba 2,N6-disubstituted adenine nucleosides as highly potent and selective A3 adenosine receptor agonists. *Journal of medicinal chemistry*, 2005, 48 (6), 1745-58.

[298] Melman, A; Gao, ZG; Kumar, D; Wan, TC; Gizewski, E; Auchampach, JA; Jacobson, KA. Design of (N)-methanocarba adenosine 5'-uronamides as species-independent A3 receptor-selective agonists. *Bioorganic & medicinal chemistry letters*, 2008, 18 (9), 2813-9.

[299] Tosh, DK; Chinn, M; Yoo, LS; Kang, DW; Luecke, H; Gao, ZG; Jacobson, KA. 2-Dialkynyl derivatives of (N)-methanocarba nucleosides: 'Clickable' A(3) adenosine receptor-selective agonists. *Bioorganic & medicinal chemistry*, 2010, 18 (2), 508-17.

[300] Tosh, DK; Chinn, M; Ivanov, AA; Klutz, AM; Gao, ZG; Jacobson, KA. Functionalized congeners of A3 adenosine receptor-selective nucleosides containing a bicyclo[3.1.0]hexane ring system. *Journal of medicinal chemistry*, 2009, 52 (23), 7580-92.

[301] Paoletta, S; Tosh, DK; Finley, A; Gizewski, ET; Moss, SM; Gao, ZG; Auchampach, JA; Salvemini, D; Jacobson, KA. Rational design of sulfonated A3 adenosine receptor-selective nucleosides as pharmacological tools to study chronic neuropathic pain. *Journal of medicinal chemistry*, 2013, 56 (14), 5949-63.

[302] Tosh, DK; Finley, A; Paoletta, S; Moss, SM; Gao, ZG; Gizewski, ET; Auchampach, JA; Salvemini, D; Jacobson, KA. In vivo phenotypic screening for treating chronic neuropathic pain: modification of C2-arylethynyl group of conformationally constrained A3 adenosine receptor agonists. *Journal of medicinal chemistry*, 2014, 57 (23), 9901-14.

[303] Melman, A; Wang, B; Joshi, BV; Gao, ZG; Castro, S; Heller, CL; Kim, SK; Jeong, LS; Jacobson, KA. Selective A(3) adenosine receptor antagonists derived from nucleosides containing a bicyclo[3.1.0]hexane ring system. *Bioorganic & medicinal chemistry*, 2008, 16 (18), 8546-56.

[304] Wan, TC; Tosh, DK; Du, L; Gizewski, ET; Jacobson, KA; Auchampach, JA. Polyamidoamine (PAMAM) dendrimer conjugate specifically activates the A3 adenosine receptor to improve post-ischemic/ reperfusion function in isolated mouse hearts. *BMC pharmacology*, 2011, 11, 11.

[305] Tosh, DK; Yoo, LS; Chinn, M; Hong, K; Kilbey, SM., 2nd; Barrett, MO; Fricks, IP; Harden, TK; Gao, ZG; Jacobson, KA. Polyamidoamine (PAMAM) dendrimer conjugates of "clickable" agonists of the A3 adenosine receptor and coactivation of the P2Y14 receptor by a tethered nucleotide. *Bioconjugate chemistry*, 2010, 21 (2), 372-84.

[306] Beukers, MW; Chang, LC; von Frijtag Drabbe Kunzel, JK; Mulder-Krieger, T; Spanjersberg, RF; Brussee, J; AP, IJ. New, non-adenosine, high-potency agonists for the human adenosine A2B receptor with an improved selectivity profile compared to the reference agonist N-ethylcarboxamidoadenosine. *Journal of medicinal chemistry*, 2004, 47 (15), 3707-9.

[307] Linden, J; Patel, A; Earl, CQ; Craig, RH; Daluge, SM. 125I-labeled 8-phenylxanthine derivatives: antagonist radioligands for adenosine A1 receptors. *Journal of medicinal chemistry*, 1988, 31 (4), 745-51.

[308] Kim, HO; Ji, XD; Melman, N; Olah, ME; Stiles, GL; Jacobson, KA. Selective ligands for rat A3 adenosine receptors: structure-activity relationships of 1,3-dialkylxanthine 7-riboside derivatives. *Journal of medicinal chemistry*, 1994, 37 (23), 4020-30.

[309] Linden, J; Thai, T; Figler, H; Jin, X; Robeva, AS. Characterization of human A(2B) adenosine receptors: radioligand binding, western blotting, and coupling to G(q) in human embryonic kidney 293 cells and HMC-1 mast cells. *Molecular pharmacology*, 1999, 56 (4), 705-13.

[310] Priego, EM; von Frijtag Drabbe Kuenzel, J; AP, IJ; Camarasa, MJ; Perez-Perez, MJ. Pyrido[2,1-f]purine-2,4-dione derivatives as a novel class of highly potent human A(3) adenosine receptor antagonists. *Journal of medicinal chemistry*, 2002, 45 (16), 3337-44.

[311] Priego, EM; Perez-Perez, MJ; von Frijtag Drabbe Kuenzel, JK; de Vries, H; Ijzerman, AP; Camarasa, MJ; Martin-Santamaria, S. Selective human adenosine A3 antagonists based on pyrido[2,1-f]purine-2,4-diones: novel features of hA3 antagonist binding. *ChemMedChem*, 2008, 3 (1), 111-9.

[312] Baraldi, PG; Preti, D; Tabrizi, MA; Fruttarolo, F; Romagnoli, R; Zaid, NA; Moorman, AR; Merighi, S; Varani, K; Borea, PA. New pyrrolo[2,1-f]purine-2,4-dione and imidazo[2,1-f]purine-2,4-dione derivatives as potent and selective human A3 adenosine receptor antagonists. *Journal of medicinal chemistry*, 2005, 48 (14), 4697-701.

[313] Baraldi, PG; Preti, D; Tabrizi, MA; Romagnoli, R; Saponaro, G; Baraldi, S; Botta, M; Bernardini, C; Tafi, A; Tuccinardi, T; Martinelli, A; Varani, K; Borea, PA. Structure-activity relationship studies of a new series of imidazo[2,1-f]purinones as potent and

selective A(3) adenosine receptor antagonists. *Bioorganic & medicinal chemistry*, 2008, 16 (24), 10281-94.

[314] Muller, CE; Thorand, M; Qurishi, R; Diekmann, M; Jacobson, KA; Padgett, WL; Daly, JW. Imidazo[2,1-i]purin-5-ones and related tricyclic water-soluble purine derivatives: potent A(2A)- and A(3)-adenosine receptor antagonists. *Journal of medicinal chemistry*, 2002, 45 (16), 3440-50.

[315] Ozola, V; Thorand, M; Diekmann, M; Qurishi, R; Schumacher, B; Jacobson, KA; Muller, CE. 2-Phenylimidazo[2,1-i]purin-5-ones: structure-activity relationships and characterization of potent and selective inverse agonists at Human A3 adenosine receptors. *Bioorganic & medicinal chemistry*, 2003, 11 (3), 347-56.

[316] Saki, M; Tsumuki, H; Nonaka, H; Shimada, J; Ichimura, M. KF26777 (2-(4-bromophenyl)-7,8-dihydro-4-propyl-1H-imidazo[2,1-i]purin-5(4H)   -one dihydrochloride), a new potent and selective adenosine A3 receptor antagonist. *European journal of pharmacology*, 2002, 444 (3), 133-41.

[317] Muller, CE; Diekmann, M; Thorand, M; Ozola, V., [(3)H]8-Ethyl-4-methyl-2-phenyl-(8R)-4,5,7,8-tetrahydro-1H-imidazo[2,1-i]-purin-5 -one ([(3)H]PSB-11), a novel high-affinity antagonist radioligand for human A(3) adenosine receptors. *Bioorganic & medicinal chemistry letters*, 2002, 12 (3), 501-3.

[318] Baraldi, PG; Preti, D; Zaid, AN; Saponaro, G; Tabrizi, MA; Baraldi, S; Romagnoli, R; Moorman, AR; Varani, K; Cosconati, S; Di Maro, S; Marinelli, L; Novellino, E; Borea, PA. New 2-heterocyclyl-imidazo[2,1-i]purin-5-one derivatives as potent and selective human A3 adenosine receptor antagonists. *Journal of medicinal chemistry*, 2011, 54 (14), 5205-20.

[319] Francis, JE; Cash, WD; Psychoyos, S; Ghai, G; Wenk, P; Friedmann, RC; Atkins, C; Warren, V; Furness, P; Hyun, JL; et al. Structure-activity profile of a series of novel triazoloquinazoline adenosine antagonists. *Journal of medicinal chemistry*, 1988, 31 (5), 1014-20.

[320] Kim, YC; Ji, XD; Jacobson, KA. Derivatives of the triazoloquinazoline adenosine antagonist (CGS15943) are selective for the human A3 receptor subtype. *Journal of medicinal chemistry*, 1996, 39 (21), 4142-8.

[321] Okamura, T; Kurogi, Y; Hashimoto, K; Nishikawa, H; Nagao, Y. Facile synthesis of fused 1,2,4-triazolo[1,5-c]pyrimidine derivatives as human adenosine A3 receptor ligands. *Bioorganic & medicinal chemistry letters*, 2004, 14 (10), 2443-6.

[322] Kozma, E; Kumar, TS; Federico, S; Phan, K; Balasubramanian, R; Gao, ZG; Paoletta, S; Moro, S; Spalluto, G; Jacobson, KA. Novel fluorescent antagonist as a molecular probe in A(3) adenosine receptor binding assays using flow cytometry. *Biochemical pharmacology*, 2012, 83 (11), 1552-61.

[323] Baraldi, PG; Cacciari, B; Romagnoli, R; Spalluto, G; Klotz, KN; Leung, E; Varani, K; Gessi, S; Merighi, S; Borea, PA. Pyrazolo[4,3-e]-1,2,4-triazolo[1,5-c]pyrimidine derivatives as highly potent and selective human A(3) adenosine receptor antagonists. *Journal of medicinal chemistry*, 1999, 42 (22), 4473-8.

[324] Baraldi, PG; Cacciari, B; Romagnoli, R; Spalluto, G; Moro, S; Klotz, KN; Leung, E; Varani, K; Gessi, S; Merighi, S; Borea, PA. Pyrazolo[4,3-e]1,2,4-triazolo[1,5-c]pyrimidine derivatives as highly potent and selective human A(3) adenosine receptor antagonists: influence of the chain at the N(8) pyrazole nitrogen. *Journal of medicinal chemistry*, 2000, 43 (25), 4768-80.

[325] Baraldi, PG; Cacciari, B; Moro, S; Spalluto, G; Pastorin, G; Da Ros, T; Klotz, KN; Varani, K; Gessi, S; Borea, PA. Synthesis, biological activity, and molecular modeling investigation of new pyrazolo[4,3-e]-1,2,4-triazolo[1,5-c]pyrimidine derivatives as human A(3) adenosine receptor antagonists. *Journal of medicinal chemistry*, 2002, 45 (4), 770-80.

[326] Maconi, A; Pastorin, G; Da Ros, T; Spalluto, G; Gao, ZG; Jacobson, KA; Baraldi, PG; Cacciari, B; Varani, K; Moro, S; Borea, PA. Synthesis, biological properties, and molecular modeling investigation of the first potent, selective, and water-soluble human A(3) adenosine receptor antagonist. *Journal of medicinal chemistry*, 2002, 45 (17), 3579-82.

[327] Pastorin, G; Da Ros, T; Bolcato, C; Montopoli, C; Moro, S; Cacciari, B; Baraldi, PG; Varani, K; Borea, PA; Spalluto, G. Synthesis and biological studies of a new series of 5-heteroarylcarbamoylaminopyrazolo[4,3-e]1,2,4-triazolo[1,5-c]pyrimidines as human A3 adenosine receptor antagonists. Influence of the heteroaryl substituent on binding affinity and molecular modeling investigations. *Journal of medicinal chemistry*, 2006, 49 (5), 1720-9.

[328] Varani, K; Merighi, S; Gessi, S; Klotz, KN; Leung, E; Baraldi, PG; Cacciari, B; Romagnoli, R; Spalluto, G; Borea, PA. [(3)H]MRE 3008F20: a novel antagonist radioligand for the pharmacological and biochemical characterization of human A(3) adenosine receptors. *Molecular pharmacology*, 2000, 57 (5), 968-75.

[329] Cheong, SL; Dolzhenko, A; Kachler, S; Paoletta, S; Federico, S; Cacciari, B; Dolzhenko, A; Klotz, KN; Moro, S; Spalluto, G; Pastorin, G. The significance of 2-furyl ring substitution with a 2-(para-substituted) aryl group in a new series of pyrazolo-triazolo-pyrimidines as potent and highly selective hA(3) adenosine receptors antagonists: new insights into structure-affinity relationship and receptor-antagonist recognition. *Journal of medicinal chemistry*, 2010, 53 (8), 3361-75.

[330] Federico, S; Ciancetta, A; Sabbadin, D; Paoletta, S; Pastorin, G; Cacciari, B; Klotz, KN; Moro, S; Spalluto, G. Exploring the directionality of 5-substitutions in a new series of 5-alkylaminopyrazolo[4,3-e]1,2,4-triazolo[1,5-c]pyrimidine as a strategy to design novel human a(3) adenosine receptor antagonists. *Journal of medicinal chemistry*, 2012, 55 (22), 9654-68.

[331] Okamura, T; Kurogi, Y; Hashimoto, K; Sato, S; Nishikawa, H; Kiryu, K; Nagao, Y. Structure-activity relationships of adenosine A3 receptor ligands: new potential therapy for the treatment of glaucoma. *Bioorganic & medicinal chemistry letters*, 2004, 14 (14), 3775-9.

[332] Colotta, V; Catarzi, D; Varano, F; Cecchi, L; Filacchioni, G; Martini, C; Trincavelli, L; Lucacchini, A. Synthesis and structure-activity relationships of a new set of 2-arylpyrazolo[3,4-c]quinoline derivatives as adenosine receptor antagonists. *Journal of medicinal chemistry*, 2000, 43 (16), 3118-24.

[333] Colotta, V; Catarzi, D; Varano, F; Filacchioni, G; Martini, C; Trincavelli, L; Lucacchini, A. Synthesis and structure-activity relationships of a new set of 1,2,4-triazolo[4,3-a]quinoxalin-1-one derivatives as adenosine receptor antagonists. *Bioorganic & medicinal chemistry*, 2003, 11 (16), 3541-50.

[334] Colotta, V; Catarzi, D; Varano, F; Calabri, FR; Lenzi, O; Filacchioni, G; Martini, C; Trincavelli, L; Deflorian, F; Moro, S. 1,2,4-triazolo[4,3-a]quinoxalin-1-one moiety as an attractive scaffold to develop new potent and selective human A3 adenosine receptor

antagonists: synthesis, pharmacological, and ligand-receptor modeling studies. *Journal of medicinal chemistry*, 2004, 47 (14), 3580-90.

[335] Lenzi, O; Colotta, V; Catarzi, D; Varano, F; Filacchioni, G; Martini, C; Trincavelli, L; Ciampi, O; Varani, K; Marighetti, F; Morizzo, E; Moro, S. 4-amido-2-aryl-1,2,4-triazolo[4,3-a]quinoxalin-1-ones as new potent and selective human A3 adenosine receptor antagonists. synthesis, pharmacological evaluation, and ligand-receptor modeling studies. *Journal of medicinal chemistry*, 2006, 49 (13), 3916-25.

[336] Colotta, V; Catarzi, D; Varano, F; Lenzi, O; Filacchioni, G; Martini, C; Trincavelli, L; Ciampi, O; Traini, C; Pugliese, AM; Pedata, F; Morizzo, E; Moro, S. Synthesis, ligand-receptor modeling studies and pharmacological evaluation of novel 4-modified-2-aryl-1,2,4-triazolo[4,3-a]quinoxalin-1-one derivatives as potent and selective human A3 adenosine receptor antagonists. *Bioorganic & medicinal chemistry*, 2008, 16 (11), 6086-102.

[337] Vernall, AJ; Stoddart, LA; Briddon, SJ; Hill, SJ; Kellam, B. Highly potent and selective fluorescent antagonists of the human adenosine A(3) receptor based on the 1,2,4-triazolo[4,3-a]quinoxalin-1-one scaffold. *Journal of medicinal chemistry*, 2012, 55 (4), 1771-82.

[338] Catarzi, D; Colotta, V; Varano, F; Calabri, FR; Lenzi, O; Filacchioni, G; Trincavelli, L; Martini, C; Tralli, A; Montopoli, C; Moro, S. 2-aryl-8-chloro-1,2,4-triazolo[1,5-a]quinoxalin-4-amines as highly potent A1 and A3 adenosine receptor antagonists. *Bioorganic & medicinal chemistry*, 2005, 13 (3), 705-15.

[339] Catarzi, D; Colotta, V; Varano, F; Lenzi, O; Filacchioni, G; Trincavelli, L; Martini, C; Montopoli, C; Moro, S. 1,2,4-Triazolo[1,5-a]quinoxaline as a versatile tool for the design of selective human A3 adenosine receptor antagonists: synthesis, biological evaluation, and molecular modeling studies of 2-(hetero)aryl- and 2-carboxy-substituted derivatives. *Journal of medicinal chemistry*, 2005, 48 (25), 7932-45.

[340] Colotta, V; Catarzi, D; Varano, F; Capelli, F; Lenzi, O; Filacchioni, G; Martini, C; Trincavelli, L; Ciampi, O; Pugliese, AM; Pedata, F; Schiesaro, A; Morizzo, E; Moro, S. New 2-arylpyrazolo[3,4-c]quinoline derivatives as potent and selective human A3 adenosine receptor antagonists. Synthesis, pharmacological evaluation, and ligand-receptor modeling studies. *Journal of medicinal chemistry*, 2007, 50 (17), 4061-74.

[341] Baraldi, PG; Tabrizi, MA; Preti, D; Bovero, A; Fruttarolo, F; Romagnoli, R; Zaid, NA; Moorman, AR; Varani, K; Borea, PA. New 2-arylpyrazolo[4,3-c]quinoline derivatives as potent and selective human A3 adenosine receptor antagonists. *Journal of medicinal chemistry*, 2005, 48 (15), 5001-8.

[342] Colotta, V; Lenzi, O; Catarzi, D; Varano, F; Filacchioni, G; Martini, C; Trincavelli, L; Ciampi, O; Pugliese, AM; Traini, C; Pedata, F; Morizzo, E; Moro, S. Pyrido[2,3-e]-1,2,4-triazolo[4,3-a]pyrazin-1-one as a new scaffold to develop potent and selective human A3 adenosine receptor antagonists. Synthesis, pharmacological evaluation, and ligand-receptor modeling studies. *Journal of medicinal chemistry*, 2009, 52 (8), 2407-19.

[343] Da Settimo, F; Primofiore, G; Taliani, S; Marini, AM; La Motta, C; Simorini, F; Salerno, S; Sergianni, V; Tuccinardi, T; Martinelli, A; Cosimelli, B; Greco, G; Novellino, E; Ciampi, O; Trincavelli, ML; Martini, C. 5-amino-2-phenyl[1,2,3]triazolo[1,2-a][1,2,4]benzotriazin-1-one: a versatile scaffold to obtain

potent and selective A3 adenosine receptor antagonists. *Journal of medicinal chemistry*, 2007, 50 (23), 5676-84.

[344] Colotta, V; Catarzi, D; Varano, F; Cecchi, L; Filacchioni, G; Martini, C; Trincavelli, L; Lucacchini, A. 1,2,4-Triazolo[4,3-a]quinoxalin-1-one: a versatile tool for the synthesis of potent and selective adenosine receptor antagonists. *Journal of medicinal chemistry*, 2000, 43 (6), 1158-64.

[345] Gao, M; Gao, AC; Wang, M; Zheng, QH. Simple synthesis of new carbon-11-labeled 1,2,4-triazolo[4,3-a]quinoxalin-1-one derivatives for PET imaging of A(3) adenosine receptor. *Applied radiation and isotopes : including data, instrumentation and methods for use in agriculture, industry and medicine*, 2014, 91, 71-8.

[346] Ji, XD; Melman, N; Jacobson, KA. Interactions of flavonoids and other phytochemicals with adenosine receptors. *Journal of medicinal chemistry*, 1996, 39 (3), 781-8.

[347] Karton, Y; Jiang, JL; Ji, XD; Melman, N; Olah, ME; Stiles, GL; Jacobson, KA. Synthesis and biological activities of flavonoid derivatives as A3 adenosine receptor antagonists. *Journal of medicinal chemistry*, 1996, 39 (12), 2293-301.

[348] Moro, S; van Rhee, AM; Sanders, LH; Jacobson, KA. Flavonoid derivatives as adenosine receptor antagonists: a comparison of the hypothetical receptor binding site based on a comparative molecular field analysis model. *Journal of medicinal chemistry*, 1998, 41 (1), 46-52.

[349] Jacobson, KA; Moro, S; Manthey, JA; West, PL; Ji, XD. Interactions of flavones and other phytochemicals with adenosine receptors. *Advances in experimental medicine and biology*, 2002, 505, 163-71.

[350] (a) Matos, MJ; Gaspar, A; Kachler, S; Klotz, KN; Borges, F; Santana, L; Uriarte, E. Targeting adenosine receptors with coumarins: synthesis and binding activities of amide and carbamate derivatives. *The Journal of pharmacy and pharmacology*, 2013, 65 (1), 30-4. (b) Matos, MJ; Hogger, V; Gaspar, A; Kachler, S; Borges, F; Uriarte, E; Santana, L; Klotz, KN. Synthesis and adenosine receptors binding affinities of a series of 3-arylcoumarins. *The Journal of pharmacy and pharmacology*, 2013, 65 (11), 1590-7. (c) Matos, MJ; Vilar, S; Kachler, S; Fonseca, A; Santana, L; Uriarte, E; Borges, F; Tatonetti, NP; Klotz, KN. Insight into the interactions between novel coumarin derivatives and human A3 adenosine receptors. *ChemMedChem*, 2014, 9 (10), 2245-53.

[351] van Muijlwijk-Koezen, JE; Timmerman, H; Link, R; van der Goot, H; AP, IJ. A novel class of adenosine A3 receptor ligands. 1. 3-(2-Pyridinyl)isoquinoline derivatives. *Journal of medicinal chemistry*, 1998, 41 (21), 3987-93.

[352] van Muijlwijk-Koezen, JE; Timmerman, H; Link, R; van der Goot, H; Ijzerman, AP. A novel class of adenosine A3 receptor ligands. 2. Structure affinity profile of a series of isoquinoline and quinazoline compounds. *Journal of medicinal chemistry*, 1998, 41 (21), 3994-4000.

[353] van Muijlwijk-Koezen, JE; Timmerman, H; van der Goot, H; Menge, WM; Frijtag Von Drabbe Kunzel, J; de Groote, M; AP, IJ. Isoquinoline and quinazoline urea analogues as antagonists for the human adenosine A(3) receptor. *Journal of medicinal chemistry*, 2000, 43 (11), 2227-38.

[354] Gao, ZG; Van Muijlwijk-Koezen, JE; Chen, A; Muller, CE; Ijzerman, AP; Jacobson, KA. Allosteric modulation of A(3) adenosine receptors by a series of 3-(2-pyridinyl)isoquinoline derivatives. *Molecular pharmacology*, 2001, 60 (5), 1057-63.

[355] Morizzo, E; Capelli, F; Lenzi, O; Catarzi, D; Varano, F; Filacchioni, G; Vincenzi, F; Varani, K; Borea, PA; Colotta, V; Moro, S. Scouting human A3 adenosine receptor antagonist binding mode using a molecular simplification approach: from triazoloquinoxaline to a pyrimidine skeleton as a key study. *Journal of medicinal chemistry*, 2007, 50 (26), 6596-606.

[356] Poli, D; Catarzi, D; Colotta, V; Varano, F; Filacchioni, G; Daniele, S; Trincavelli, L; Martini, C; Paoletta, S; Moro, S. The identification of the 2-phenylphthalazin-1(2H)-one scaffold as a new decorable core skeleton for the design of potent and selective human A3 adenosine receptor antagonists. *Journal of medicinal chemistry*, 2011, 54 (7), 2102-13.

[357] Lenzi, O; Colotta, V; Catarzi, D; Varano, F; Poli, D; Filacchioni, G; Varani, K; Vincenzi, F; Borea, PA; Paoletta, S; Morizzo, E; Moro, S. 2-Phenylpyrazolo[4,3-d]pyrimidin-7-one as a new scaffold to obtain potent and selective human A3 adenosine receptor antagonists: new insights into the receptor-antagonist recognition. *Journal of medicinal chemistry*, 2009, 52 (23), 7640-52.

[358] Squarcialupi, L; Colotta, V; Catarzi, D; Varano, F; Filacchioni, G; Varani, K; Corciulo, C; Vincenzi, F; Borea, PA; Ghelardini, C; Di Cesare Mannelli, L; Ciancetta, A; Moro, S. 2-Arylpyrazolo[4,3-d]pyrimidin-7-amino derivatives as new potent and selective human A3 adenosine receptor antagonists. Molecular modeling studies and pharmacological evaluation. *Journal of medicinal chemistry*, 2013, 56 (6), 2256-69.

[359] Taliani, S; La Motta, C; Mugnaini, L; Simorini, F; Salerno, S; Marini, AM; Da Settimo, F; Cosconati, S; Cosimelli, B; Greco, G; Limongelli, V; Marinelli, L; Novellino, E; Ciampi, O; Daniele, S; Trincavelli, ML; Martini, C. Novel N2-substituted pyrazolo[3,4-d]pyrimidine adenosine A3 receptor antagonists: inhibition of A3-mediated human glioblastoma cell proliferation. *Journal of medicinal chemistry*, 2010, 53 (10), 3954-63.

[360] Biagi, G; Bianucci, AM; Coi, A; Costa, B; Fabbrini, L; Giorgi, I; Livi, O; Micco, I; Pacchini, F; Santini, E; Leonardi, M; Nofal, FA; Salerni, OL; Scartoni, V. 2,9-disubstituted-N6-(arylcarbamoyl)-8-azaadenines as new selective A3 adenosine receptor antagonists: synthesis, biochemical and molecular modelling studies. *Bioorganic & medicinal chemistry*, 2005, 13 (15), 4679-93.

[361] Klotz, KN; Kachler, S; Lambertucci, C; Vittori, S; Volpini, R; Cristalli, G. 9-Ethyladenine derivatives as adenosine receptor antagonists: 2- and 8-substitution results in distinct selectivities. *Naunyn-Schmiedeberg's archives of pharmacology*, 2003, 367 (6), 629-34.

[362] Volpini, R; Costanzi, S; Lambertucci, C; Vittori, S; Martini, C; Trincavelli, ML; Klotz, KN; Cristalli, G. 2- and 8-alkynyl-9-ethyladenines: Synthesis and biological activity at human and rat adenosine receptors. *Purinergic signalling*, 2005, 1 (2), 173-81.

[363] Perreira, M; Jiang, JK; Klutz, AM; Gao, ZG; Shainberg, A; Lu, C; Thomas, CJ; Jacobson, KA. "Reversine" and its 2-substituted adenine derivatives as potent and selective A3 adenosine receptor antagonists. *Journal of medicinal chemistry*, 2005, 48 (15), 4910-8.

[364] Gao, ZG; Joshi, BV; Klutz, AM; Kim, SK; Lee, HW; Kim, HO; Jeong, LS; Jacobson, KA. Conversion of A3 adenosine receptor agonists into selective antagonists by modification of the 5'-ribofuran-uronamide moiety. *Bioorganic & medicinal chemistry letters*, 2006, 16 (3), 596-601.

[365] Pal, S; Choi, WJ; Choe, SA; Heller, CL; Gao, ZG; Chinn, M; Jacobson, KA; Hou, X; Lee, SK; Kim, HO; Jeong, LS. Structure-activity relationships of truncated adenosine derivatives as highly potent and selective human A3 adenosine receptor antagonists. *Bioorganic & medicinal chemistry*, 2009, 17 (10), 3733-8.

[366] Lee, J; Hwang, I; Lee, JH; Lee, HW; Jeong, LS; Ha, H. The selective A3AR antagonist LJ-1888 ameliorates UUO-induced tubulointerstitial fibrosis. *The American journal of pathology*, 2013, 183 (5), 1488-97.

[367] Nayak, A; Chandra, G; Hwang, I; Kim, K; Hou, X; Kim, HO; Sahu, PK; Roy, KK; Yoo, J; Lee, Y; Cui, M; Choi, S; Moss, SM; Phan, K; Gao, ZG; Ha, H; Jacobson, KA; Jeong, LS. Synthesis and anti-renal fibrosis activity of conformationally locked truncated 2-hexynyl-N(6)-substituted-(N)-methanocarba-nucleosides as A3 adenosine receptor antagonists and partial agonists. *Journal of medicinal chemistry*, 2014, 57 (4), 1344-54.

[368] Auchampach, JA; Gizewski, ET; Wan, TC; de Castro, S; Brown, GG. Jr; Jacobson, KA. Synthesis and pharmacological characterization of [(125)I]MRS5127, a high affinity, selective agonist radioligand for the A3 adenosine receptor. *Biochemical pharmacology*, 2010, 79 (7), 967-73.

[369] Kiesewetter, DO; Lang, L; Ma, Y; Bhattacharjee, AK; Gao, ZG; Joshi, BV; Melman, A; de Castro, S; Jacobson, KA. Synthesis and characterization of [76Br]-labeled high-affinity A3 adenosine receptor ligands for positron emission tomography. *Nuclear medicine and biology*, 2009, 36 (1), 3-10.

[370] Ravn, J; Qvortrup, K; Rosenbohm, C; Koch, T. Design, synthesis, and biological evaluation of LNA nucleosides as adenosine A3 receptor ligands. *Bioorganic & medicinal chemistry*, 2007, 15 (16), 5440-7.

[371] van Rhee, AM; Jiang, JL; Melman, N; Olah, ME; Stiles, GL; Jacobson, KA. Interaction of 1,4-dihydropyridine and pyridine derivatives with adenosine receptors: selectivity for A3 receptors. *Journal of medicinal chemistry*, 1996, 39 (15), 2980-9.

[372] Jiang, J; van Rhee, AM; Chang, L; Patchornik, A; Ji, XD; Evans, P; Melman, N; Jacobson, KA. Structure-activity relationships of 4-(phenylethynyl)-6-phenyl-1,4-dihydropyridines as highly selective A3 adenosine receptor antagonists. *Journal of medicinal chemistry*, 1997, 40 (16), 2596-608.

[373] Li, AH; Moro, S; Melman, N; Ji, XD; Jacobson, KA. Structure-activity relationships and molecular modeling of 3, 5-diacyl-2,4-dialkylpyridine derivatives as selective A3 adenosine receptor antagonists. *Journal of medicinal chemistry*, 1998, 41 (17), 3186-201.

[374] Cosimelli, B; Greco, G; Ehlardo, M; Novellino, E; Da Settimo, F; Taliani, S; La Motta, C; Bellandi, M; Tuccinardi, T; Martinelli, A; Ciampi, O; Trincavelli, ML; Martini, C. Derivatives of 4-amino-6-hydroxy-2-mercaptopyrimidine as novel, potent, and selective A3 adenosine receptor antagonists. *Journal of medicinal chemistry*, 2008, 51 (6), 1764-70.

[375] Yaziji, V; Rodriguez, D; Gutierrez-de-Teran, H; Coelho, A; Caamano, O; Garcia-Mera, X; Brea, J; Loza, MI; Cadavid, MI; Sotelo, E. Pyrimidine derivatives as potent and selective A3 adenosine receptor antagonists. *Journal of medicinal chemistry*, 2011, 54 (2), 457-71.

[376] Jung, KY; Kim, SK; Gao, ZG; Gross, AS; Melman, N; Jacobson, KA; Kim, YC. Structure-activity relationships of thiazole and thiadiazole derivatives as potent and

selective human adenosine A3 receptor antagonists. *Bioorganic & medicinal chemistry*, 2004, 12 (3), 613-23.

[377] Press, NJ; Keller, TH; Tranter, P; Beer, D; Jones, K; Faessler, A; Heng, R; Lewis, C; Howe, T; Gedeck, P; Mazzoni, L; Fozard, JR. New highly potent and selective adenosine A(3) receptor antagonists. *Current topics in medicinal chemistry*, 2004, 4 (8), 863-70.

[378] Miwatashi, S; Arikawa, Y; Matsumoto, T; Uga, K; Kanzaki, N; Imai, YN; Ohkawa, S. Synthesis and biological activities of 4-phenyl-5-pyridyl-1,3-thiazole derivatives as selective adenosine A3 antagonists. *Chemical & pharmaceutical bulletin*, 2008, 56 (8), 1126-37.

In: Pharmaceutical Formulation
Editor: Bruce Moore

ISBN: 978-1-63484-082-8
© 2015 Nova Science Publishers, Inc.

Chapter 2

DEVELOPMENT OF NEW ENZYME INHIBITORS: PURINE BIOISOSTERE PERSPECTIVE

Felicia Phei Lin Lim, Anna V. Dolzhenko and Anton V. Dolzhenko

School of Pharmacy, Monash University Malaysia
School of Pharmacy, Curtin Health Innovation Research Institute,
Curtin University, Australia

ABSTRACT

This chapter focuses on concepts of isosterism and bioisosterism in modern medicinal chemistry. Drug design and development aspects are illustrated by applying these concepts to the construction of potent enzyme inhibitors. Particular attention is devoted to bioisosteric modifications of the purine scaffold contributing to the molecular diversity and improvements of pharmacodynamic and pharmacokinetic parameters of compounds. The scope of this chapter covers heterocyclic systems generated by various aza- / deaza- replacements of the purine ring atoms. The success of the bioisosterism strategy in the development of clinically useful enzyme inhibitors, constructed on the purine related heterocyclic systems, is exemplified by several important drugs. Sildenafil, inhibiting cGMP-specific phosphodiesterase type 5, has been a blockbuster drug since its launch to the market. It was followed by further isosteric modifications of the ring system that resulted in the development of another representative of this class, vardenafil. Allopurinol, inhibiting one of the key purine catabolizing enzymes – xanthine oxidase, has been a gold standard of chronic gout therapy for more than 50 years. Examples of other drugs, drug candidates, and lead compounds are also discussed in the context of recent trends in the enzyme inhibitor research.

INTRODUCTION

In drug discovery, the categories of drug targets encompasses enzymes, G-protein coupled receptors (GPCRs), nuclear hormone receptors, ion channels, transporters, and nucleic acids [1, 2]. The overall distribution of druggable targets show enzymes dominating with 47% followed by GPCRs accounting for 30% and the remaining categories representing less than a quarter of drug targets [3]. Enzymes function as biological catalysts promoting multi-step biochemical reactions that allow to achieve remarkable rate accelerations by matching protein and substrate chemical groups in transition state [1, 2]. By taking advantage of the catalytic chemistry of enzymes, inhibitors offer unique opportunities in the area of drug design making them a special class of drug target. Many marketed enzyme inhibitors are structurally similar to their enzyme substrate [1, 2]. The design of enzyme inhibitors containing a structural motif related to the substrate has been an effective strategy in the drug discovery program. One type of examples includes bioisosteric modifications of the purine scaffold.

Purine is an N-containing heterocyclic system, which is the core structure of adenine and guanine in RNA and DNA [4]. Purine nucleotides (ATP, GTP, cAMP, cGMP, NAD, FAD) act as co-factors, substrates or mediators in the functioning of many proteins [4, 5]. Protein kinases are enzymes carrying out the phosphorylation of ATP [6], while cyclic nucleotide phosphodiesterases (PDE) are enzymes hydrolyzing cAMP and cGMP [7]. The purine catabolism also involves different enzymes in various pathways all leading up to the generation of end-product, which is uric acid in humans and allantoin in many mammals (Figure 1) [8]. Irreversible deamination of adenosine to inosine is carried out by adenosine deaminase (ADA) [9], while the ubiquitous purine nucleoside phosphorylase (PNP) is responsible for the inter-conversion between (deoxy)nucleosides and bases [10]. With the exception of adenosine, PNP catalyzes (in the presence of inorganic phosphate) the reversible cleavage of N-ribosidic bonds of purine nucleosides, such as inosine and guanosine, to generate ribose 1-phosphate and corresponding purine bases (hypoxanthine and guanine) [10]. Guanine deaminase is responsible for the hydrolytic deamination of guanine to xanthine [11]. The oxidative hydroxylation of hypoxanthine catalyzed by xanthine oxidase (XO) produces xanthine, which is consequently oxidized by the same enzyme to uric acid [12]. Urate oxidase (UO), an enzyme present in many mammals excluding humans and higher primates, is responsible for converting highly insoluble uric acid into 5-hydroxyisourate which can be further degraded into allantoin for excretion [13].

The abovementioned enzymes are valuable drug targets for many drug discovery programs. Most notable are the kinases, which represent the largest category of potentially novel clinical trial drug targets: 145 unique kinases are identified as targets of established and clinical trial agents and 64% of them are potentially new targets not directed by approved pharmaceuticals [14].

The majority of clinical trials for PDE inhibitors are FDA-approved drugs undergoing phase IV for additional efficacy data. However, there are a substantial amount of novel PDE inhibitors which are currently being investigated in trials for the treatment of diseases for which PDE inhibitors have been already proved to be effective therapies [15].

Various aza- /deaza- replacements of carbon/nitrogen atoms in the purine ring have been successfully employed in the design and development of the enzyme inhibitors. This chapter will focus on the success of the bioisosterism strategy in the development of enzyme inhibitors: inhibitors of important kinases, PDEs, and purine catabolizing enzymes (ADA, PNP, XO and UO) based on the purine related heterocyclic systems.

USING PURINE ISOSTERIC SCAFFOLDS IN THE DEVELOPMENT OF KINASE INHIBITORS

Kinases regulate multiple important cellular activities through protein phosphorylation. These activities include signalling, transcription, metabolism and cell cycle progression [16]. More than 500 protein kinases have been identified from the human genome sequence [17] and they represent approximately 20% of the druggable genome [18]. This promising group of enzymes have been the focus of intensive investigations in the drug discovery field with hundreds of drug candidates undergoing clinical trials. Over the past decade, 30 kinase targeting drugs have been approved for clinical use, mainly as anti-cancer agents [19]. In an estimated 50-70% current oncology drug discovery programs, protein kinase inhibitors served as main targets [19].

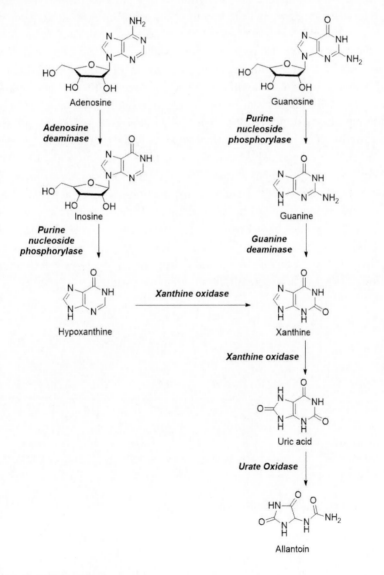

Figure 1. Purine catabolism pathway.

As regulators of cell division cycle, cyclin-dependent kinases (CDKs) are a family of enzymes that have raised considerable interest in the field of oncology [20-23]. Developing new CDK inhibitors appears to be a promising avenue for the search of novel anticancer agents. One of the first investigated scaffolds for the development of CDK inhibitors was the purine heterocyclic system leading to the discovery of roscovitine (**1**) (Figure 2) [24-26], which is currently undergoing clinical trials as an anticancer agent. The success of roscovitine inspired further explorations oriented towards the design of purine isosteres through redistribution of nitrogen atoms around the purine scaffold. Moving the nitrogen from position 9 to position 5 of roscovitine led to the development of potent CDK2 inhibitor **2** [25]. This isosteric modification to the pyrazolo[1,5-*a*][1,3,5]triazine scaffold maintained similar conformations and binding modes to CDK2 in addition to comparable pharmacokinetic profiles to roscovitine [25]. Nonetheless, compound **2** had more than 5 times improvement in CDK inhibitory activity compared to roscovitine [25]. Compound **2** was also about 14 times more potent than roscovitine when tested by the National Cancer Institute against panel of 60 tumor cell lines (NCI60), with no partiality towards any specific form of tumor [26]. Additionally, an improved *in vitro* bioactivity of **2** was seen in the Ewing's sarcoma xenograft mouse model system whereby the dose needed for **2** (25 mg/kg) was half of that for roscovitine (50 mg/kg) to achieve similar outcome (more than 70% of tumor inhibition) [26].

A different isosteric modification of roscovitine with switching the nitrogen atom position in the purine scaffold from 9 to 8 led to another potent CDK2 inhibitor **3** with the pyrazolo[4,3-*d*]pyrimidine core [27]. Comparable binding modes were observed between roscovitine and **3**, but compound **3** demonstrated better efficiency in the CDK inhibition compared to roscovitine [27]. When tested against a panel of human cell lines representing a range of tumour types, compound **3** showed distinctively stronger activity than roscovitine. Compound **3** and roscovitine were also evaluated against NCI60 and compound **3** demonstrated about two times higher overall activity compared to roscovitine [27].

Additionally, cell cycle analysis for both compound **3** and roscovitine showed similar patterns of cell-cycle blockade, but compound **3** arrested cell cycle for two human cancer cell lines (MCF-7 and RPMI-8226) more efficiently than roscovitne.

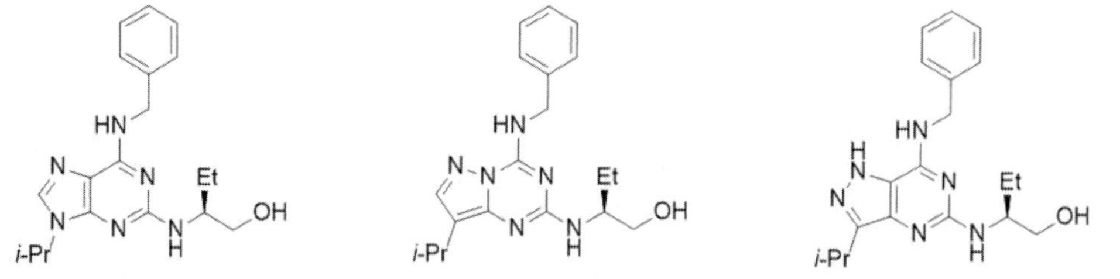

1, (*R*)-roscovitine
IC_{50} = 0.15 µM (CDK2/CYCE),
0.22 µM (CDK2/CYCA)

2
IC_{50} = 0.026 µM (CDK2/CYCE),
0.04 µM (CDK2/CYCA)

3
IC_{50} = 0.04 µM (CDK2/CYCE)

Figure 2. CDK inhibitors based on purine isosteric scaffolds.

Another kinase important in the oncology area is casein kinase II (CK2), a highly conserved protein serine/threonine kinase which has been shown to be overexpressed in human cancers [28, 29]. CK2 is involved in cell proliferation, transformation, senescence and apoptosis [28, 29]. The pyrazolo[1,5-*a*][1,3,5]triazine core has proven to be suitable for the development of new potent CK2 inhibitors (Figure 3). Substituted 2,4-diaminopyrazolo[1,5-*a*][1,3,5]triazines (**4-6**) showed good CK2 inhibition, which in turn translated into *in vitro* antiproliferative activity against prostate (PC3) and colon (HCT116) cancer cell lines [30, 31]. Although macrocyclic compound **5** had a decrease in CK inhibition compared to **4**, there was almost ten times improvement in anticancer activity [31]. Improved cellular activity for macrocyclic compound **5** was attributed to its increase in membrane permeability. Modification of structure to a more complex substituted arylamino moiety in position 4 resulted in structure **6** with improved CK2 inhibitory potency, better aqueous solubility and increased activity against both PC3 and HCT116 cell lines [31].

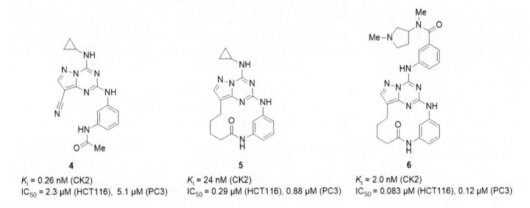

4
K_i = 0.26 nM (CK2)
IC_{50} = 2.3 µM (HCT116), 5.1 µM (PC3)

5
K_i = 24 nM (CK2)
IC_{50} = 0.29 µM (HCT116), 0.88 µM (PC3)

6
K_i = 2.0 nM (CK2)
IC_{50} = 0.083 µM (HCT116), 0.12 µM (PC3)

Figure 3. 5-Aza-9-deazapurine based inhibitors of CK2.

Aurora kinases family, which encompass Aurora-A, -B and -C, also belongs to the group of serine/threonine kinases. These kinases play a pivotal role in different stages of cell cycle and are overexpressed in a range of human malignancies [32, 33]. Thus, Aurora kinases have gained prominence as anticancer targets. There is still ongoing clinical evaluation for the ideal inhibitor profile in relation to isoform selectivity with majority of developed Aurora kinase inhibitors exerting their effect on all three isoforms [34-36]. Selective inhibitors will be useful for detailed functional studies of each isoform of this kinase family.

In the high throughput screening (HTS) against recombinant human Aurora-A kinase, a hit compound with the imidazo[4,5-*b*]pyridine scaffold was identified [37]. This 1-deazapurine core served as a useful template for the generation of lead compound **7**, a potent inhibitor of Aurora kinase (Figure 4). From these encouraging results, a medicinal chemistry program was initiated with the aim to convert compound **7** into an orally bioavailable inhibitor of Aurora kinase suitable for pre-clinical evaluation. To avoid the potential toxicophore liabilities associated with compound **7**, a new class of imidazo[4,5-*b*]pyridine-based Aurora kinase inhibitors was developed with a common 1-benzylpiperazinyl motif at position 7 [38]. Subsequently, the physicochemical property refinement by the introduction of solubilizing groups to reduce liphophilicity led to the developent of compound **8** [38]. *In vivo* efficacy testing showed that following oral administration, compound **8** inhibited the growth of SW620 colon cancer cell xenografts with no perceived toxicities. However, compound **8** had showed inhibition against antitarget hERG ion-channel (IC_{50} = 3.0 µM) and low human liver microsomal stability with 86% metabolized after 30 minutes incubation thus, potentially limiting its preclinical development [38]. The attempts to identify Aurora kinase inhibitors with higher metabolic stability and wider safety margin against hERG were continued using compound **8** as the starting point with the aim to find an orally bioavailable preclinical development candidate. Replacing (4-methylpiperazin-1-yl)phenyl with five membered heteroaromatics led to the discovery of ideal 1,3-dimethyl-1H-pyrazol-4-yl substituent at C-2 [39]. Consequent property refinement of substituents gave compound **9**, a dual FMS-like receptor tyrosine kinase-3 (FLT3)/Aurora kinase inhibitor which is orally bioavailable and displays high selectivity within the tested kinome [39]. Besides Aurora kinase inhibition, compound **9** was found to significantly inhibit mutant FLT3 kinases including FLT3-ITD. This particular mutant causes constitutive FLT3 kinase activation detectable in acute myeloid leukaemia (AML) within 20-35% of adults and 15% of children and conferring a poor prognosis in both age groups. Compound **9** has been selected as a preclinical development candidate for the treatment of cancers, particularly AML in adults and children who are becoming resistant to existing therapies [39]. Advancing from the initial success, the imidazo[4,5-*b*]pyridine scaffold was further explored in the search for new highly selective Aurora-A kinase inhibitors. From a library of imidazo[4,5-*b*]pyridine derivatives, compounds **10a,b** were selected due to their high selectivity for inhibition of Aurora-A over Aurora-B in both biochemical assays and cell-based assays using Hela cervical cancer and HCT 116 human colon carcinoma cells [40]. These compounds could serve as valuable small molecule tools for further exploration of Aurora-A function in cells.

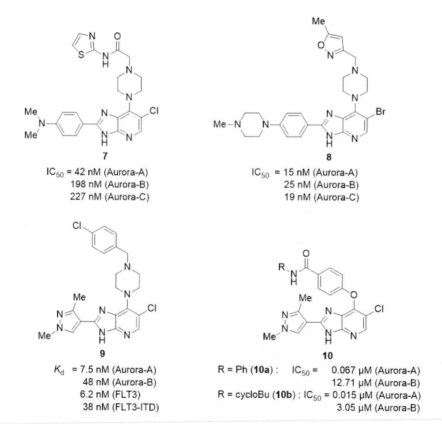

Figure 4. 1-Deazapurine based inhibitors of Aurora kinases.

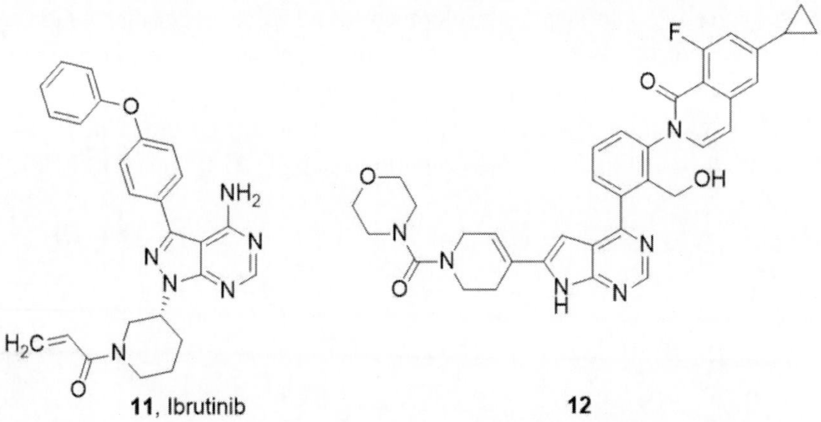

Figure 5. BTK inhibitors based on purine isosteric scaffolds.

Bruton's tyrosine kinase (BTK) belongs to the Tec family of kinases and is one of the non-receptor tyrosine kinase. Expressed mostly in hematopoietic cells, BTK plays a critical role in the signalling pathways downstream of the B-cell receptor and FcγRIIa, FcγRIIIa and FcεRI receptors [41-43]. BTK represents an intriguing drug target for the treatment of autoimmune diseases [44, 45] and B-cell malignancies [46, 47]. The active research programs on small molecules inhibiting BTK were carried out by pharmaceutical companies and eventually led to the recent approval of 8-aza-7-deazapurine derivative, ibrutinib (11) (Figure 5) for the treatment of mantle cell lymphoma (MCL) and chronic lymphocytic leukaemia (CLL) [48].

A novel class of pyrrolo[2,3-*d*]pyrimidine-based BTK inhibitors were recently explored and the most promising compound 12 showed nanomolar activity in the BTK enzyme assay [49].

Janus kinase (JAK) also a family of non-receptor tyrosine kinases comprises of four members: JAK1, JAK2, JAK3, and Tyk2, which name was originally derived from identification as just another kinase and tyrosine kinase 2. These kinases interact with signal transducer and activator of transcription (STAT) proteins through the JAK-STAT pathway and hence mediating cytokine receptor signalling [50]. The inhibition of JAK could provide an avenue for modulating cytokine-mediated effects with JAK inhibitors as potential therapeutic agents for certain cancers and inflammatory diseases [50].

Two 7-deazapurine-based JAK inhibitors, ruxolitinib (13) [51] and tofacitinib (14) [52] have been recently approved for the treatment of myeloproliferative disorders and psoriasis, respectively (Figure 6). Ruxolitinib is currently undergoing clinical trials for the treatment of acute leukaemia [53], pancreatic cancer [54], breast cancer [55], Hodgkin's Lymphoma [56] and polycythemia vera [57] while tofacitinib is being investigated for the treatment of rheumatoid arthritis [58] and alopecia [59].

Baricitinib (15), a JAK1/JAK2 inhibitor developed by Incyte and Eli Lilly, is currently in Phase III clinical trials for the treatment of rheumatoid arthritis [60].

Another non-receptor tyrosine kinase, activated Cdc42-associated tyrosine kinase 1 (ACK1) has been recently investigated in the search for new anticancer agents. Poor prognosis is seen when ACK1 gene is amplified in primary tumours, thus inhibition of ACK1 represents an interesting approach in development of new anticancer therapeutic agents [61]. Purine and its aza- / deaza- isosteres were interesting templates in the pursuit for new ACK1 inhibitors. Compound **16** with the purine scaffold exhibited micromolar ACK1 inhbition, however, through relocation of nitrogen from position 7 to 5, four times increased in potency was achieved for the resulting 5-aza-7-deazapurine analogue **17** (Figure 7).

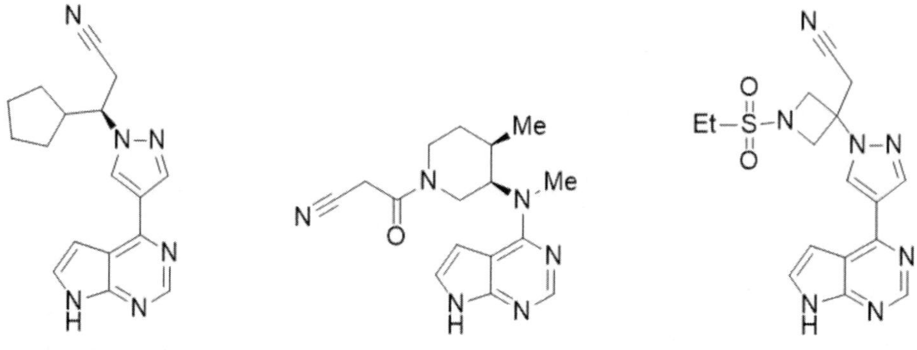

13, Ruxolitinib **14**, Tofacitinib **15**, Baricitinib

Figure 6. 7-Deazapurine based inhibitors of JAK.

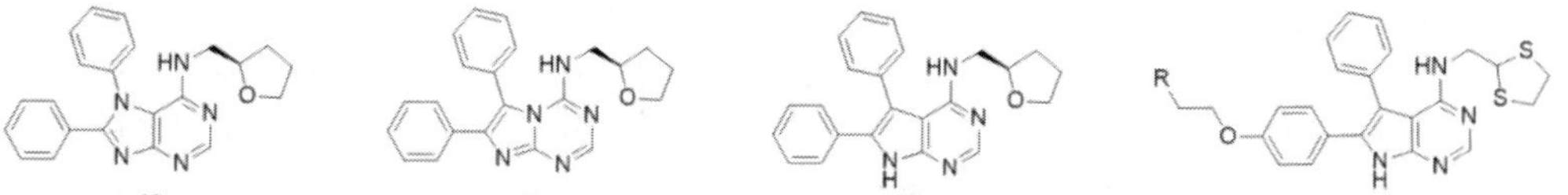

16 K_i = 7.3 μM; **17** K_i = 1.8 μM; **18** K_i = 0.006 μM; **19** R = $(CH_2)_4NH$ (**19a**) ; R = $(CH_3)_2NH$ (**19b**) : K_i = 0.0003 μM

Figure 7. Purine and its isosteres as scaffolds for ACK1 inhibitors.

Gratifyingly, elimination of nitrogen at position 7 of the purine scaffold gave pyrrolo[2,3-*d*]pyrimidine **18**, with ACK1 inhibition in the nanomolar range. The potency of **18** was more than a thousand times higher compared to the parent purine compound **16** [62]. Fine tuning the SAR for this new class of ACK1 inhibitors with the pyrrolo[2,3-*d*]pyrimidine scaffold revealed that tetrahydrofuran ring can be effectively replaced by the 1,3-dithiolane. Compounds **19a**,**b** were identified as the most potent ACK1 inhibitors in the series. *In vitro* metabolic studies show higher stability for the pyrrolidine-substituted **19a** in rat hepatocytes relative to the dimethylamine derivative **19b** [62].

The Src family kinases (SFKs) represent a group of non-receptor tyrosine kinases that encompass Blk, Fgr, Fyn, Hck, Lck, Lyn, Src, Yes and Yrk. SFKs regulate a diverse spectrum of cellular processes such as cell growth, adhesion, differentiation, migration and survival [63]. An abnormal SFK signalling is often seen in many cancers making SFK inhibitors a possible avenue for the anticancer therapeutic intervention [64, 65]. Several small molecules inhibiting SFKs have been designed based on the purine isosteric scaffold. Pyrazolo[3,4-*d*]pyrimidine derivatives **20a** (PP1) and **20b** (PP2), which can be considered as isosteric modifications of substituted adenine, were identified as selective and active in nanomolar concentrations SFK inhibitors of Lck and Fyn enzymes (Figure 8). When tested against other

SFK members, PP1 was also found to display inhibitory activity against Src and Hck kinase [66, 67].

Norvatis found that a diphenyl-substituted pyrazolo[3,4-*d*]pyrimidine **21** (CGP191) inhibited Src in micromolar concentration, however changing the scaffold to the isosteric 7-deazapurine system led to a five-fold increase in potency of 7,9-diphenyl-7-deazaadenine (**22**, CGP62464). From compound **22**, SAR-guided modifications afforded more potent Src inhibitor CGP77675 (**23**), which also showed inhibition on other SFKs such as Lck and Yes in osteoporosis and cancer models [68-71]. Another 7-deazapurine (pyrrolo[2,3-*d*]pyrimidine) derivative A-419259 (**24**) was found to be a highly selective SFK inhibitor, which was active in nanomolar concentrations against Src, Lck and Lyn enzymes [72].

A genetic link between Parkinson's disease (PD) and leucine rich repeat kinase 2 (LRRK2) has been established by genome-wide association studies. G2019S, the most prevalent LRRK2 mutation is found in both familial and sporadic PD cases [73-75]. An increase in kinase activity was observed in case of the G2019S mutation, which could lead to activation of the neuronal death signal pathway [73-75]. Hence, LRRK2 inhibitors were proposed to be potentially useful for the treatment of PD. Additionally, LRRK2 inhibitors are being actively pursued to serve as pharmacological tools for the investigation into the pathophysiological roles of LRRK2.

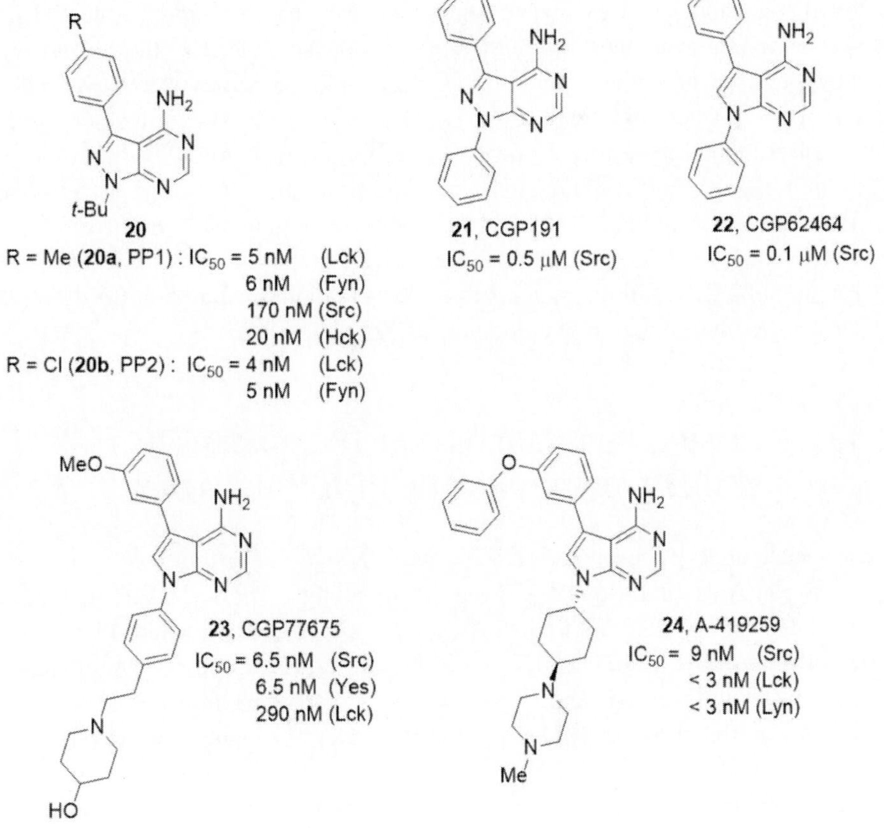

20

R = Me (**20a**, PP1) : IC$_{50}$ = 5 nM   (Lck)
                                  6 nM   (Fyn)
                              170 nM (Src)
                               20 nM (Hck)
R = Cl (**20b**, PP2) : IC$_{50}$ = 4 nM   (Lck)
                                  5 nM   (Fyn)

21, CGP191
IC$_{50}$ = 0.5 μM (Src)

22, CGP62464
IC$_{50}$ = 0.1 μM (Src)

23, CGP77675
IC$_{50}$ = 6.5 nM (Src)
         6.5 nM (Yes)
         290 nM (Lck)

24, A-419259
IC$_{50}$ = 9 nM   (Src)
        < 3 nM (Lck)
        < 3 nM (Lyn)

Figure 8. Adenine isosteres as scaffolds for SFK inhibitors.

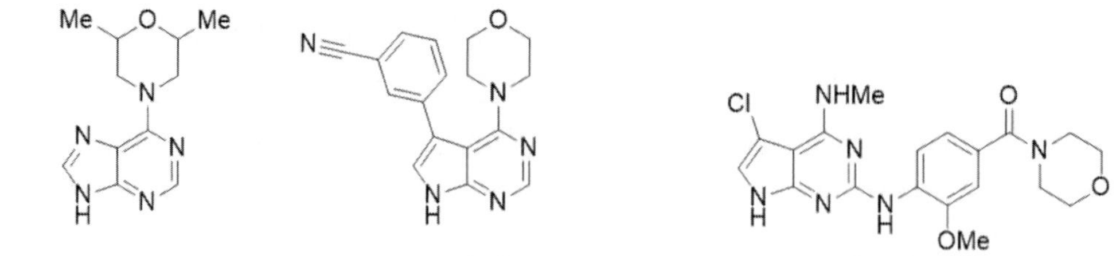

25
IC$_{50}$ = 1240 nM (LRRK2)

26
IC$_{50}$ = 3 nM (LRRK2)

27, JH-II-127
IC$_{50}$ = 6.6 nM (LRRK2-wild-type)
2.2 nM (LRRK2-G2019S)

Figure 9. Purine and its 7-deaza-isostere as scaffolds for LRRK2 inhibitors.

In the search for novel LRRK2 inhibitors, a HTS was conducted and dimethylmorpholino substituted purine **25**, was identified as a key hit at the preliminary stage (Figure 9) [76]. On the basis of hit **25**, it was found that by removing a nitrogen at position 7 of the purine scaffold, compounds with the 7-deazapurine (pyrrolo[2,3-*d*]pyrimidine) core provided a higher level of potency towards LRRK2 and further optimization lead to the development of compound **26**, which was 400 times more effective in the LRRK2 inhibition compared to **25** [76]. *In vivo* experiments demonstrated that compound **26** possessed good availability in rat with close to equal distribution across brain compartments [76]. Further testing in rodent pharmacodynamic model and two-week toxicological assessment was conducted however, higher species pharmacokinetic properties were not suitable for the advancement of compound **26** to clinical studies. Nonetheless, its overall properties were favourable for its use as a tool for further investigation of LRRK2. The successful utilization of a purine isostere template fuelled the efforts to further develop potent pyrrolo[2,3-*d*]pyrimidine-based LRRK2 inhibitors with favourable pharmacokinetic properties. 2-Anilino-4-methylamino-5-chloropyrrolo[2,3-*d*]pyrimidine, JH-II-127 (**27**) showed potent and selective inhibition of both wild-type and G2019S mutant LRRK2 [77]. Compound **27** also inhibited Ser935 phosphorylation of LRRK2 in the mouse brain after oral administration at the 30 mg/kg dose [77]. Further *in vivo* investigation of compound **27** are underway.

USING PURINE ISOSTERIC SCAFFOLDS IN THE DEVELOPMENT OF PDE INHIBITORS

Cyclic nucleotide phosphodiesterase (PDE) hydrolyses intracellular secondary messengers cyclic AMP and cyclic GMP to corresponding AMP and GMP nucleotides [78]. Currently, 11 families of PDE are known (PDE1 to PDE11) among which PDE5, PDE6 and PDE9 are cGMP-specific; PDE4, PDE7 and PDE8 are cAMP-specific. The remaining PDEs are non-specific to both cAMP and cGMP. Each of these isozymes has diverse structural properties and contributes to the regulation of intracellular messenger level in different tissues and organs [79].

Natural xanthine alkaloids caffeine (**28**), theobromine (**29**), and theophylline (**30**) and their synthetic alkylxanthine analogues 3-isobutyl-1-methylxanthine (IBMX) (**31**), enprofylline (**32**) and pentoxifylline (**33**) have long been known as non-selective PDE inhibitors and their pharmacological effects were mainly attributed to the PDE inhibition

(Figure 10) [80]. Although effective in their role as PDE inhibitors, the common drawback of these compounds is the unfavourable adverse effect profile due to non-selective interaction with a range of PDEs and other targets. Thus, selective targeting of PDE has been addressed in drug discovery and development programs to avoid or at least minimise potential side effects from the non-specific PDE inhibition.

Zaprinast (**34**) was one of the first selective PDE5 inhibitors achieved the clinical trial stage (Figure 11) [81]. Based on the 8-azaxanthine scaffold, this compound (**34**) initiated an extensive search for PDE inhibitors among heterocyclic systems resembling purine core.

Many research programs on the development of PDE inhibitors skyrocket after the approval granted in 1998 for the blockbuster drug, PDE5 inhibitor based on the 8-aza-9-deazahypoxanthine scaffold, sildenafil (**35**). It was followed by its ring isosteric modification vardenafil (**36**), which was approved for the same therapeutic application *viz.* the treatment of erectile dysfunction [82]. The commercial success of these drugs intensified PDE research centered around purine isosteres.

A group from SK chemicals (South Korea) investigated the SAR of sildenafil analogues and compounds **37-39** were identified as potent PDE5 inhibitors [83-85]. Compound **37** demonstrated good PDE5 inhibition but was less potent compared to sildenafil [83]. Exploring the SAR of pyrazolo[3,4-*d*]pyrimidines, it was found that the replacement of piperazine by piperidine connected *via* various length linkages with a carboxylic group gave a series of compounds with increased potency compared to sildenafil. The most potent PDE5 inhibitor identified in this series was compound **38** with the piperidine moiety linked *via* an ethylenic bridge to a carboxylic group mimicking the phosphate moiety of cGMP [84]. Replacement of the piperidine sulphonamide with anilinoamides yielded compound **39**, which possessed PDE5 inhibitory activity comparable with that of sildenafil [85].

Another detailed investigation of hypoxanthine derivatives and their isosteric scaffolds was carried out by Bayer AG to identify potent and selective PDE5 inhibitors [86]. Compound **40** with the hypoxanthine skeleton showed inhibition of PDE5 in nanomolar concentrations and good selectivity over PDE1 [86]. The relocation of one of the purine skeleton nitrogen atoms from position 9 to 8 and fine tuning of the substituents around the scaffold afforded compound **41**, a sildenafil analogue with triple the selectivity and almost double the potency towards PDE5 compared to the hypoxanthine derivative **40** but less potent compared to sildenafil [86, 87]. Changing the position of one nitrogen atom in compound **41** and addition of the piperazine sulphonamide moiety afforded sildenafil analogue with the 8-aza-7-deazahypoxanthine scaffold, compound **42**, which possessed higher potency and selectivity compared to **41** and the PDE5 inhibitory profile similar to sildenafil [86].

Another series of sildenafil analogues was investigated through modifications at the N-terminal sulphonamide moiety by replacement of the N-methylpiperazine moiety but maintaining the pyrazolo[3,4-*d*]pyrimidine scaffold of sildenafil. Compound **43**, demonstrating greater PDE5 inhibitory activity compared to sildenafil, was the most potent in the series [87]. Additionally, compound **43** showed better efficacy in *in vivo* testing (conscious rabbit model) than the standard drug, sildenafil [88].

The phosphodiesterase 9 (PDE9) is another recently characterized cGMP specific enzyme, which shows the greatest affinity to cGMP compared to all PDE families known to date [89]. PDE9 is insensitive up to 100 μM amongst most reference inhibitors including IBMX (**31**). PDE9 was found in various tissues including brain, kidney, spleen, colon, intestine and prostate [90]. Purine isosteres, particularly hypoxanthine scaffold analogues, have served well as a template in the search for selective PDE9 inhibitors. Thus, the 7-deaza-8-azahypoxanthine skeleton was used for the construction of BAY 73-6691 (**44**), which became the first potent and selective PDE9 inhibitor reported (Figure 12) [91]. BAY 73-6691 showed efficient penetration through cell membranes and inhibition of intracellular PDE9 when tested against PDE9 reporter cell line. Further preclinical investigations of this compound are ongoing in the course of the development of a new therapeutic agent for Alzheimer's disease [91].

28, Caffeine

29, Theobromine

30, Theophylline

31, IBMX

32, Enprofylline

33, Pentoxifylline

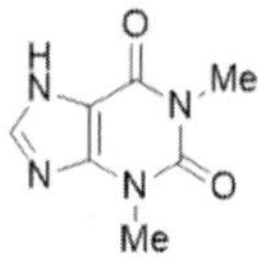

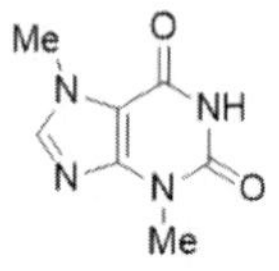

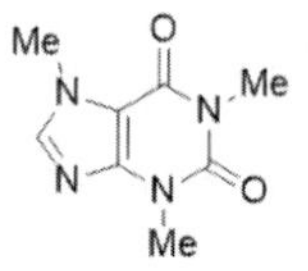

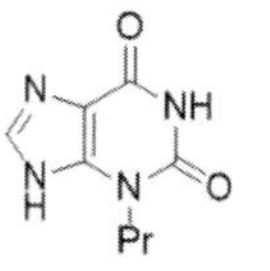

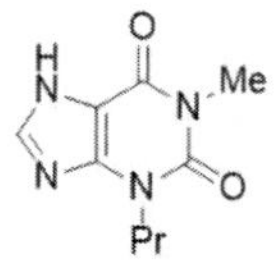

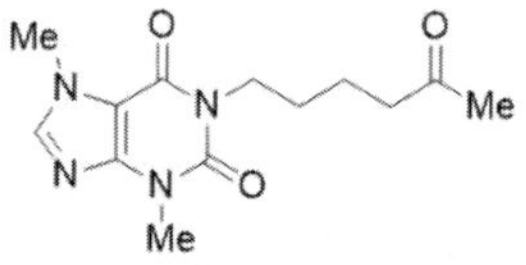

Figure 10. Non-selective purine-based PDE inhibitors.

34, Zaprinast
IC_{50} = 130 nM (PDE5)

35, Sildenafil
IC_{50} = 4-10 nM (PDE5)

36, Vardenafil
IC_{50} = 0.14-1 nM (PDE5)

37
IC_{50} = 6.25 nM (PDE5)

38
IC_{50} = 0.05 nM (PDE5)

39
IC_{50} = 0.27 nM (PDE5)

40
IC_{50} = 50 nM (PDE5)
500 nM (PDE1)

41
IC_{50} = 27 nM (PDE5)
790 nM (PDE1)

42
IC_{50} = 8 nM (PDE5)
1000 nM (PDE1)

43
IC_{50} = 1.5 nM (PDE5)

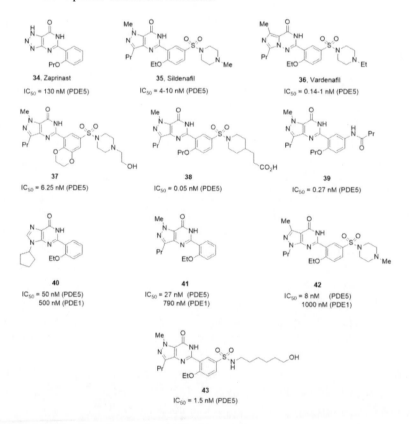

Figure 11. PDE5 inhibitors based on purine and its isosteres.

Following the initial success of BAY 73-6691, a cross-screening was conducted on representative examples from preceding PDE inhibitor programs. The 8-aza-9-deazahypoxanthine derivative **45** was identified as a potent but non-selective inhibitor of PDE9 demonstrating similar inhibitory effects on PDE1a, 1b and 1c [92]. Fine tuning of SAR gave potent and selective PDE9 inhibitors **46a,b** possessing excellent oral bioavailability. These compounds would serve as useful tools for the pharmacological investigation of PDE9 [92].

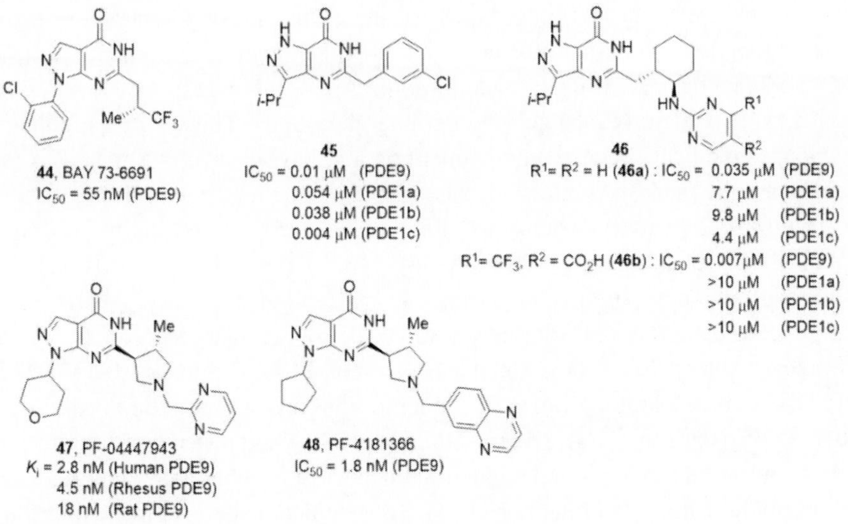

Figure 12. Purine isosteres as scaffolds for PDE9 inhibitors.

Further efforts to identify and optimize selective PDE9 inhibitors led to the discovery of PF-04447943 (**47**) constructed on the 8-aza-7-deazahypoxanthine scaffold [93, 94]. This potent and selective PDE9 inhibitor was reported to cross the blood-brain barrier enhancing rodent cognitive function after oral administration (1-10 mg/kg). Currently, development of PF-04447943 (**47**) as potential drug for the treatment of Alzheimer's disease has reached the clinical investigation stage.

Another 8-aza-7-deazahypoxanthine derivative, PF-4181366 (**48**), showed high affinity and selectivity towards PDE9, however modification of compound stereochemistry lead to a drop in PDE9 potency by almost 30 times for the less active enantiomer [95]. Compound **48** penetrated the CNS easily when dosed in rodents, and overall displayed all the attributes of a useful PDE9 pharmacological tool.

Two isogenes PDE8A and PDE8B make up one of the relatively unexplored cAMP-specific PDE8 family [96, 97]. Since its discovery, the genetic, biochemical, and pharmacological characteristics of the two PDE8s have been reported. However, their biological function and potential drugability have yet to be elucidated. A similar trait shared between PDE8 and PDE9 is the insensitivity to most PDE inhibitors including IBMX (**31**) [96, 97]. Dipyridamole, although, non-selective towards PDE8, was used experimentally to study cellular functions of PDE8 until the recent development by Pfizer the first selective PDE8 inhibitor PF-4957325 (**49**) (Figure 13) [98]. This compound (**49**) belongs to 8-azapurine (1,2,3-triazolo[4,5-*d*]pyrimidine) derivatives and has served as a breakthrough pharmacological tool for in depth studies of PDE8 functions [99]. PF-4957325 (**49**) was used to compare the steroid production in PDE8A, PDE8B, and PDE8A and B double-knockout cells [99]. From these experiments, both PDE8A and PDE8B were seen as major regulators of basal steroidogenesis.

A HTS was conducted with the aim of identifying selective inhibitors of PDE8B and one of the interesting hits was constructed using the same 8-azapurine scaffold as PF-4957325 (**49**). Optimized for greater potency, selectivity to PDE8B, and ADME properties, compound **50** demonstrated more than 1000-fold selectivity over all PDEs tested, except PDE8A. Although isoform selectivity could not be established, this highly potent and selective PDE8 inhibitor with good bioavailability advanced into the preclinical development [100].

PDE2 modulate the signalling cascade of both cAMP and cGMP and is expressed in both the central nervous system (CNS) and the peripheral systems. Thus, PDE2 regulates a range of different physiological processes and functions and have been investigated as targets for CNS, cardiovascular and respiratory diseases [101]. One of the earliest selective PDE2 inhibitor *erythro*-9-(2-hydroxy-3-nonyl)adenine (EHNA) (**51**) was initially used as a tool to explore the PDE2 pharmacology (Figure 14) [102, 103]. However, its relatively low selectivity and potency hindered further pharmacological study. Through isosteric modification of the purine scaffold, BAY-60-7550 (**52**), constructed on the imidazo[5,1-*f*][1,2,4]triazine skeleton, was developed as a potent PDE2 inhibitor. BAY-60-7550 (**52**) inhibited PDE2 in the nanomolar range of concentrations and was found to be highly selective over other PDE isoforms [104]. BAY-60-7550 (**52**) was tested in hippocampal slice preparations and rodent behavioural models and the results obtained supported the role of PDE2 inhibitors in learning and memory [104, 105]. When tested in mice using the elevated plus maze and the hole-board test, BAY-60-7550 (**52**) showed anxiolytic effects [106]. Additionally, BAY-60-7550 (**52**) reversed corticosterone-induced down-regulation of BDNF in mice thus suggesting antidepressant-like effects of the compound [107]. These results supported the potential role of PDE2 in the regulation of the stress-related cognitive impairment.

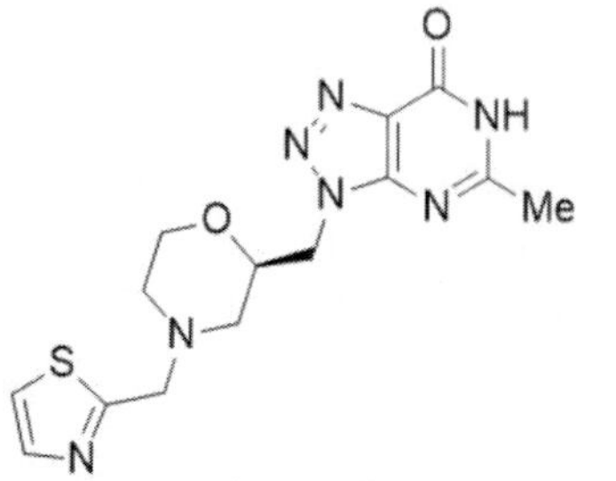

49, PF-4957325
$IC_{50} = 0.7$ nM (PDE8A)
< 1.5 nM (PDE8B)

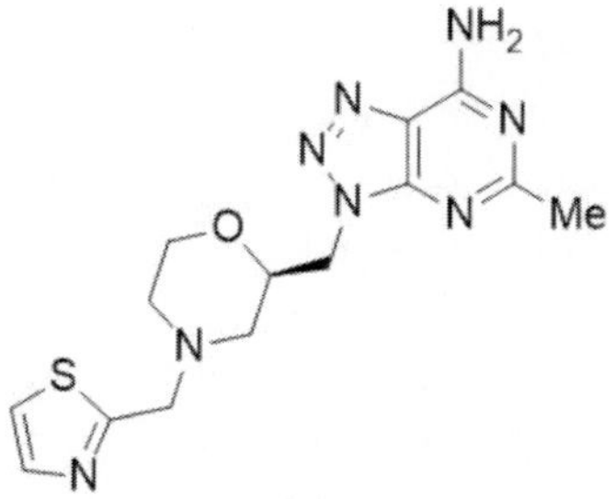

50
$IC_{50} = 1.9$ nM (PDE8A)
1.3 nM (PDE8B)

Figure 13. 8-Azapurines as scaffolds for PDE8 inhibitors.

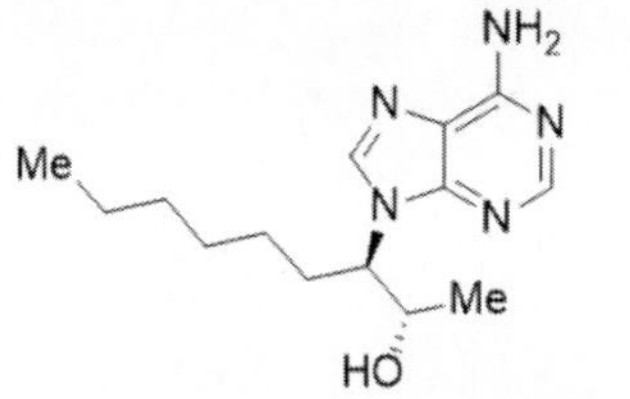

51, EHNA
K_i = 7 nM (PDE2)

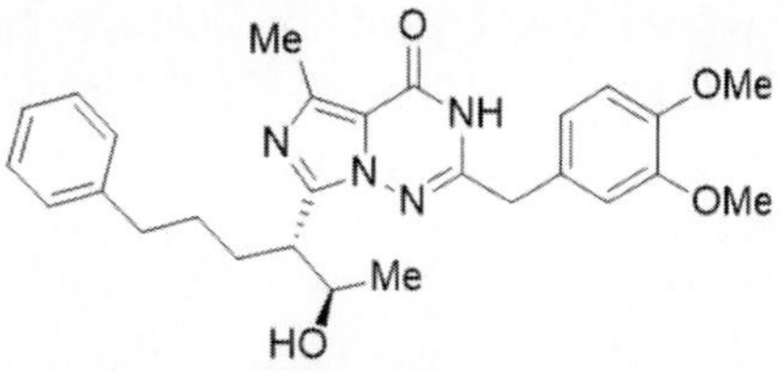

52, BAY-60-7550
IC_{50} = 2 nM (PDE2)

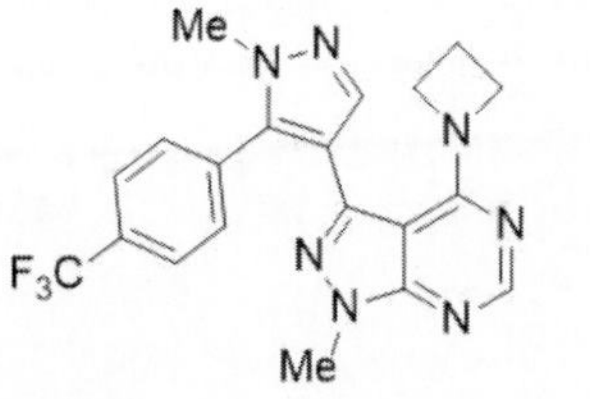

53
IC_{50} = 2 nM (PDE2)

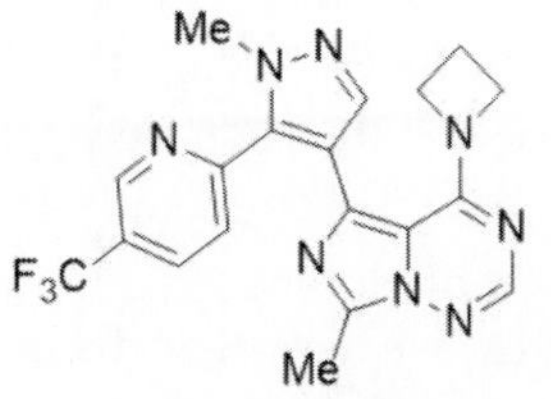

54, PF-999
IC_{50} = 1 nM (PDE2)

Figure 14. Purines and its isosteres as scaffolds for PDE2 inhibitors.

Pfizer investigated a novel series of 8-aza-7-dezapurines as PDE2 inhibitors. The lead from this series, compound **53**, displayed potent and selective PDE2 inhibition in addition to good brain permeability properties [108]. For improvement of PDE2 potency and ADME characteristics, the same research group altered the central purine affording the imidazo[5,1-*f*][1,2,4]triazine core of compound **54**, which displayed PDE2 inhibition in nanomolar concentrations [109]. This enhanced activity was postulated to stem from a more efficient interaction with the water molecules located in the catalytic domain by the nitrogen of the imidazo[5,1-*f*][1,2,4]triazine scaffold. When tested in rats, compound **54** showed efficacy in models of working memory and spatial and learning memory [110]. After further profiling, Pfizer advanced compound **54** as their clinical candidate (PF-999). In 2011, a phase I clinical trial of PF-999 (**54**) showed dose tolerance between 0.1 and 60 mg in healthy subjects. Another phase I clinical trial was completed the following year which assessed the bioavailability of a modified release formulation of PF-999 (**54**) [110].

Using Purine Isosteric Scaffolds in the Development of Purine Catabolizing Enzyme Inhibitors

Adenosine deaminase (ADA) is a purine catabolising enzyme, which irreversibly catalyses the hydrolytic degradation of adenosine and 2'-deoxyadenosine to inosine and 2'-deoxyinosine respectively [111]. ADA is ubiquitous to almost all mammalian cells and regulates both intra- and extracellular adenosine concentrations, playing a vital role in maintaining the immune system integrity [112]. ADA inhibitors have been proposed for the treatment of lymphoproliferative malignancies, cardiovascular diseases and as novel anti-inflammatory drugs [113-116]. Additionally, the pharmacological action of ADA inhibitors in preventing metabolic breakdown would be synergistic when used alongside adenosine-based antiviral and antitumor drugs [117]. Potent ADA inhibitors can be classified into ground-state inhibitors, when their structure mimics that of endogenous ADA substrate adenosine, and transition-state inhibitors, when their structures are similar to the tetrahedral transition-state intermediate.

EHNA (51), which was mentioned above as a PDE2 inhibitor, has also been reported as an ADA inhibitor with the complex mechanism of enzyme inhibition (Figure 15) [118]. The initial stage involves classical competitive inhibition of ADA followed by a consecutive rearrangement of the enzyme and inhibitor forming a tight ADA-inhibitor complex [119]. Despite high inhibitory activity against ADA, poor toxicological profile makes EHNA unsuitable for clinical use [120, 121]. To improve the unfavourable properties, the design of novel ADA inhibitors centered on modification of the purine scaffold and the development aza- / deaza- bioisosteres of purine.

Analogues of EHNA, whereby the adenine was replaced by the 8-aza-7-deazaadenine (4-aminopyrazolo[3,4-d]pyrimidine) scaffold were investigated as potential ADA inhibitors [122]. From the 1- and 2-alkyl derivatives of the 4-aminopyrazolo[3,4-d]pyrimidines synthesized and evaluated, substitution at position 2 was found to enhance ADA inhibitory activity. The increase of compound potency correlated with the extension of alkyl chain length, reaching the maximum at n-decyl substituent. From the series, (R)-isomer of compound 55 showed the highest inhibitory activity against ADA with more than 20 times greater effect than that of reference standard, EHNA [122]. Switching the stereochemistry of 55 caused a substantial drop in potency (K_i = 37.5 nM). Docking of this (S)-enantiomer of 55 in the ADA active site revealed that the molecule was pointing outside the enzyme cleft causing improper fitting of many top-ranked clusters in the active site [122]. Biological testing of compound 55 demonstrated its ability to reduce both systemic and intestinal inflammatory parameters when administered intraperitoneally to rats with colitis [123]. Additionally, both macroscopic and histological features of colonic tissues showed improvement together with a reduction in the levels of inflammatory mediators.

From the success of compound 55, further evaluation was initiated with the same purine isosteric scaffold. Modification of the C-4 amino group led to the development of 8-aza-7-deazahypoxanthines as novel ADA inhibitors [124]. The most active compound in this series 56 was significantly more potent than the purine-based reference EHNA. When tested in rats with colitis, compound 56 decreased both intestinal and systemic inflammation processes [124].

Naturally occurring purine nucleoside nebularine (57), first isolated as the principle of a press-juice from *Lepista nebularis*, is a well-known inhibitor of ADA [125, 126]. It was found that by bioisosteric changes to 8-azanebularine 58, a 400 times increase in potency was achieved [126]. This superior ADA binding affinity could be due to the presence of 8-nitrogen facilitating the formation of covalent hydrate. It was also hypothesized that hydration of these compounds across the 1,6-bond is needed to mimic the structure of the transition state during the ADA deamination of adenosine [126]. Thus, 1,6-dihydro-8-azanebularine (59) showed much weaker ADA inhibition compared to the fully aromatic 8-azanebularine due to its inability to add a water molecule to the 1,6-bond [126].

Purine nucleoside phosphorylase (PNP) is an enzyme involve in the purine salvage pathway; it catalyzes the reversible phosphorolytic cleavage of the glycosidic bond of ribo- and deoxyribonucleosides to generate ribose(deoxyribose)-1-phosphate and purine bases

[127]. In humans, PNP plays a key role in proper functioning of cellular immune systems. PNP deficiency causes impaired T-cell function with no apparent effects on B-cell function [127]. Thus, PNP inhibitors represent a new target for the development of selective immunosuppressive agents.

One of the methods for the design of novel PNP inhibitors is the transition state theory whereby a perfect match of the transition state would bind tighter compared to substrate by the factors of enzymatic rate enhancement. The application of this theory to inosine as a substrate led to the design of 9-deazanucleotide analogues, which were confirmed to be potent inhibitors of PNP. They were denoted as immucillins, from which forodesine (immucillin H) (60) became the most well-known PNP inhibitor (Figure 16) [128]. Forodesine demonstrated activity in preclinical studies with malignant cells and clinical efficiency against T-cell lymphoma and T-cell acute lymphoblastic leukaemia (T-ALL) [129, 130]. Forodesine was also proved to be effective and well-tolerated as a single agent in relapsed or refractory T-ALL. Results from the phase I clinical trial of patients with T-cell malignancies treated with forodesine demonstrated the pharmacological efficacy of this drug in elevating dGuo and intracellular dGTP in addition to antileukaemic activity [131].

Another structurally similar transition-state PNP inhibitor identified in this group is ulodesine (BCX-4208) (61), which inhibits PNP in human, mouse, rat and monkey in the nanomolar concentration range. Ulodesine is currently undergoing clinic investigations to assess its safety, tolerability, and pharmacodynamic effects after oral administration in patients with moderate to severe chronic plaque psoriasis [132].

An ongoing program on developing potent transition-state PNP inhibitors identified compound 62, a fluoro-substituted ulodesine [133]. Stereochemistry of 62 played an important role in the effective inhibition of PNP. The (3S,4S)-enantiomer 62 was found to bind more efficiently (K_i*= 0.33 nM) to PNP at lower concentration compared to ulodesine (K_i*= 1.10 nM). The racemic mixture of 62 with its enantiomer also demonstrated a good binding to PNP (K_i*= 0.50 nM). However, the (3R,4R)-enantiomer of 62 was substantially less active (K_i* = 18 nM) [133]. Despite oral bioavailability of 62 in mice at 0.2mg/kg, ADME characteristics and duration of action of 62 were less encouraging than the same parameters of ulodesine [133].

The reversible phosphorylation of purine nucleosides by PNP involves a ternary complex of enzyme, orthophosphate and nucleosides. Thus, the presence of features of both substrates (nucleosides and orthophosphate) in the structure of a compound was suggested for the design of new "multi-substrate analogue" PNP inhibitors. Halazy et al. developed one of the most potent multi-substrate PNP inhibitor, 9-(5',5'-difluoro-5'-phosphonopentyl)guanine (DFPP-G) (63) [134]. The crystallography data confirmed the binding of DFPP-G to both nucleoside and phosphate-binding sites of PNP. The putative hydrogen bonds on the base-binding site indicated a non-direct contact mediated by a water molecule which is entropically disfavoured. It was hypothesized that removal of the water molecule from the complex may induce a tighter binding to PNP. Based on these results, a new candidate, 9-(5',5'-difluoro-5'-phosphonopentyl)-9-deazaguanine (DFPP-DG) (64) was designed as a PNP inhibitor, whereby the removal of nitrogen at N-9 of the guanine base of DFPP-G gave the 9-deazaguanine bioisostere [135, 136]. The inhibitory properties of DFPP-DG, tested against calf-spleen and human erythrocyte PNPs, were found to be more prominent than those of DFPP-G [135-138]. From initial velocity experiments, the apparent inhibition constants of

DFPP-DG (K_i^{app} = 8.1 nM) proved to be more potent than those of DFPP-G (K_i^{app} = 10.8 nM) [136-138].

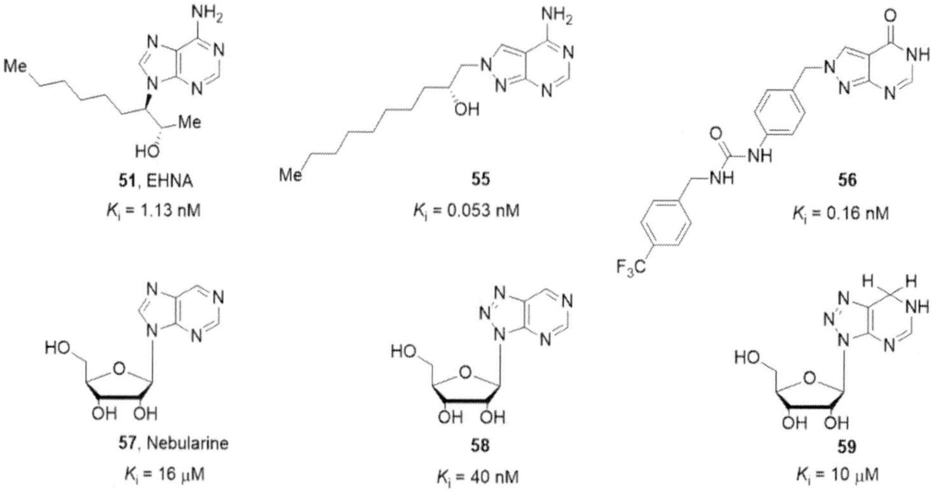

51, EHNA
K_i = 1.13 nM

55
K_i = 0.053 nM

56
K_i = 0.16 nM

57, Nebularine
K_i = 16 μM

58
K_i = 40 nM

59
K_i = 10 μM

Figure 15. ADA Inhibitors based on purine and its isosteres.

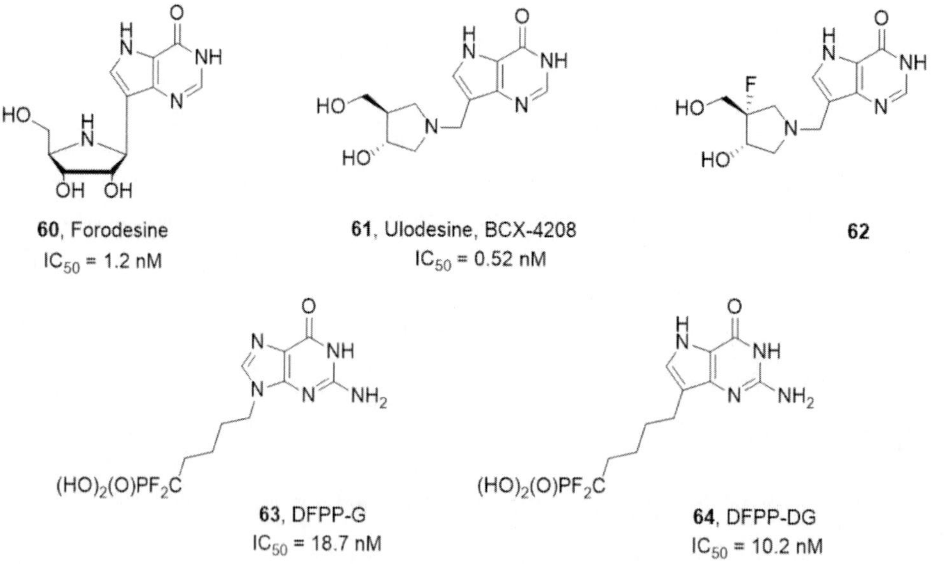

60, Forodesine
IC_{50} = 1.2 nM

61, Ulodesine, BCX-4208
IC_{50} = 0.52 nM

62

63, DFPP-G
IC_{50} = 18.7 nM

64, DFPP-DG
IC_{50} = 10.2 nM

Figure 16. PNP inhibitors based on purine and purine isosteres.

In the metabolic transformations of purines, xanthine oxidase (XO) is a key enzyme catalysing the subsequent hydroxylation of hypoxanthine and xanthine producing final product of purine catabolism, uric acid [139]. Hyperuricaemia and chronic gout can be combated through XO regulation with classical XO inhibitor, allopurinol (**65**) being the most widely prescribed uric-acid lowering agent in the gout therapy [140].

Robins et al. investigated a range of compounds with scaffolds isosteric to guanine, hypoxanthine and xanthine [141]. An isostere of hypoxanthine and allopurinol, 5-azahypoxanthine (**66**) was marginally active in XO inhibition (Figure 17). 5-Azaxanthine

(**67a**), an isostere of xanthine and oxypurinol (active allopurinol metabolite), showed slightly better XO inhibition compared to **66**, but switching to its thio-analogue **67b** caused a drop in activity. The *S*-methylation of **67b** increase XO inhibitory activity of **68b** making it more potent than allopurinol [141]. However, *O*-methylation of 5-azaxanthine (**67a**) had an opposite effect, decreasing the potency of **68a** by almost half [141].

Interesting results were obtained with compounds bearing the 5-aza-9-deazapurine (pyrazolo[1,5-*a*][1,3,5]triazine) scaffold. Based on this skeleton, bioisostere of allopurinol **69a** possessed similar XO inhibitory activity with its structural analogue **66** [141]. However, introduction of a C-7 phenyl ring to the pyrazolo[1,5-*a*][1,3,5]triazine system (**69b**) led to a dramatic increase in the XO inhibitory effect with more than three order greater activity compared to the unsubstituted **69a**. Introduction of a C-2 methyl group (**69c**) led to a significant loss of XO activity, showing intolerance to even minor structural modification at this position [141].

A very potent 5-aza-9-deazahypoxanthine-based XO inhibitor, BOF-4272 (**70**), synthesized by a Japanese research group [142, 143] displayed promising results in a number of *in vitro* and *in vivo* studies [144-146] and experiments on healthy human volunteers [147]. BOF-4272 (**70**) caused a significant reduction of XO activity by targeting the main organs for uric acid production, particularly the liver and the small intestine [148]. Additionally, BOF-4272 (**70**) prevented cell necrosis by decreasing the concentration of free radicals generated by XO [148]. The study on the mechanism of XO inhibition by BOF-4272 (**70**) [144, 145], revealed that alteration of the molecule stereochemistry changed the potency of XO inhibition. Both the (*R*)-(+)-enantiomer and (*S*)-(-) enantiomer were determined to be mixed type inhibitors with the latter having a much higher activity than the former [144, 145]. Additionally, pharmacokinetic parameters and biotransformation of BOF-4272 (**70**) were also determined by the stereochemistry of the molecule [149-151]. Thus, additional studies were conducted on the more potent asymmetrical (*S*)-(-)-BOF-4272 [152, 153]

Another purine isosteric skeleton, 8-aza-7-deazadenine, was successfully used as a template for the design and development of potent XO inhibitors. Compound **71a** was identified as a potent inhibitor of XO [154]. The glycine methyl ester was found to be the optimal substituent in the series, although replacement with a trifluormethyl (**71b**), cyano (**71c**) or nitro (**71d**) group maintained IC_{50} values close to or below 2 μM making all of them more potent than allopurinol [154].

Opening of the uric acid pyrimidine ring involves an enzymatic oxidation by urate oxidase (UO) followed by a non-enzymatic hydrolysis producing allantoin, which is 5-10 times more soluble at physiological conditions than uric acid [155].

Although absent in humans, UO is an inducible enzyme found in a variety of microorganisms including pathogens [156], where its role as a powerful scavenger of free radicals protects the pathogen during macrophage ingestion [157, 158].

Thus, blockage of UO may lead to impaired growth of pathogens. The absence of UO in humans makes this enzyme a potential drug target for the treatment of infection by pathogens [159-161] and a substantial amount of research have been focus on the understanding of the exact catalytic mechanism of this enzyme.

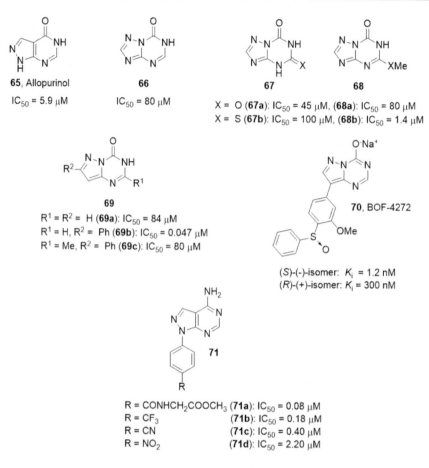

65, Allopurinol
$IC_{50} = 5.9 \mu M$

66
$IC_{50} = 80 \mu M$

67
68

X = O (**67a**): $IC_{50} = 45 \mu M$, (**68a**): $IC_{50} = 80 \mu M$
X = S (**67b**): $IC_{50} = 100 \mu M$, (**68b**): $IC_{50} = 1.4 \mu M$

69
$R^1 = R^2 = H$ (**69a**): $IC_{50} = 84 \mu M$
$R^1 = H, R^2 = Ph$ (**69b**): $IC_{50} = 0.047 \mu M$
$R^1 = Me, R^2 = Ph$ (**69c**): $IC_{50} = 80 \mu M$

70, BOF-4272

(S)-(-)-isomer: $K_i = 1.2$ nM
(R)-(+)-isomer: $K_i = 300$ nM

71

R = $CONHCH_2COOCH_3$ (**71a**): $IC_{50} = 0.08 \mu M$
R = CF_3 (**71b**): $IC_{50} = 0.18 \mu M$
R = CN   (**71c**): $IC_{50} = 0.40 \mu M$
R = NO_2 (**71d**): $IC_{50} = 2.20 \mu M$

Figure 17. Purine isosteres as scaffolds for XO inhibitors.

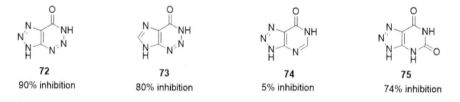

72
90% inhibition

73
80% inhibition

74
5% inhibition

75
74% inhibition

Figure 18. *In vitro* inhibition of UO by hypoxanthine and xanthine isosteres (1 x 10^{-5} M).

Analogues of hypoxanthine have shown inhibitory activity towards UO [162]. When tested *in vitro*, it was found that 2,8-diazahypoxanthine (**72**), 2-azahypoxanthine (**73**), 8-azahypoxanthine (**74**) and 8-azaxanthine (**75**) showed inhibitory activity against UO (Figure 18) [162]. A huge drop in inhibitory activity is seen with the removal of nitrogen at position 8 of the hypoxanthine molecule. However, an opposite effect is observed with xanthine as 8-azaxanthine (**75**) displayed good UO inhibitory activity. When tested on UO *in vivo*, 2,8-diazahypoxanthine (**72**), administered intraperitoneally, caused the greatest increase in uric acid levels with a concomitant decrease in allantoin levels [162]. Although showing minimal *in vitro* UO inhibition, 8-azahypoxanthine (**74**) was a strong inhibitor *in vivo*, similar with 8-azaxanthine (**75**). This could possibly be due to *in vivo* oxidation of **74** to **75**, thus correlating the potent *in vivo* and *in vitro* activity of 8-azaxanthine (**75**). On the other hand, 2-azahypoxanthine (**73**) showed no change in allantoin or uric acid levels *in vivo* although displaying strong inhibition of UO *in vitro* [162]. UO inhibitors are valuable tools used in many studies designed to investigate the functionality of the enzyme. Crystallographic studies of UO from *Aspergillus flavus* utilizes 8-azaxanthine (**75**) to investigate the relevance of the hydrophobic cavity in the catalytic mechanism [163]. 8-Azaxanthine (**75**) was also used to study different polymorphs of a recombinant UO from *Aspergillus flavus* [164]. With X-ray structures of UO and various inhibitors available, Oksanen et al. [165] used a complex of 8-azaxanthine (**75**) and UO for the collection of high-resolution X-ray and neutron diffraction data which provided vital information towards elucidating the mechanism of catalysis.

CONCLUSION

The biososterism concept applied to molecular scaffolds has been an extremely valuable strategy in the design of new therapeutic agents. In the development of enzyme inhibitors, modification of purine to its isosteric analogues expands chemical space and often gave improved pharmacokinetic and pharmacodynamics properties favoring pre-clinical and clinical selection.

Compounds bearing the purine isosteric scaffolds have been proven to be effective in targeting enzymes involved in the transformations of purine-based biomolecules. Investigation around various aza-/deaza-purines were successful in the development of inhibitors of various kinases, PDEs, and enzymes involved in the purine catabolism (ADA, PNP, XO, and UO). Well-known blockbuster drugs such as XO inhibitor, allopurinol and PDE5 inhibitors, sildenafil and vardenafil are remarkable illustrations of these accomplishments. Purine bioisosteres contributed to the recent boom in the field of kinase inhibitors by the approval of BTK inhibitor, ibrutinib and JAK inhibitors, ruxolitinib and tofacitinib, which have been taking their niche in the pharmaceutical market, and many more purine bioisosteres in pre-clinical and clinical development stages.

REFERENCES

[1]   Robertson, JG. Mechanistic basis of enzyme-targeted drugs. *Biochemistry*, 2005, *44* (15), 5561-5571.

[2]   Robertson, JG. Enzymes as a special class of therapeutic target: clinical drugs and modes of action. *Curr. Opin. Struct. Biol.* 2007, *17* (6), 674-679.

[3]   Hopkins, AL; Groom, CR. Opinion: The druggable genome. *Nat. Rev. Drug Discovery*, 2002, *1* (9), 727-730.

[4]   Legraverend, M; Grierson, DS. The purines: Potent and versatile small molecule inhibitors and modulators of key biological targets. *Bioorg. Med. Chem.* 2006, *14* (12), 3987-4006.

[5]   Murray, JM; Bussiere, DE. Targeting the purinome. *Methods Mol. Biol.* 2009, *575*, 47-92.

[6]   Russo, GL; Russo, M; Ungaro, P. AMP-activated protein kinase: A target for old drugs against diabetes and cancer. *Biochem. Pharmacol.* 2013, *86* (3), 339-350.

[7]   Perry, MJ; Higgs, GA. Chemotherapeutic potential of phosphodiesterase inhibitors. *Curr. Opin. Chem. Biol.* 1998, *2* (4), 472-481.

[8]   Werner, AK; Witte, CP. The biochemistry of nitrogen mobilization: purine ring catabolism. *Trends Plant Sci.* 2011, *16* (7), 381-387.

[9]   Cristalli, G; Costanzi, S; Lambertucci, C; Lupidi, G; Vittori, S; Volpini, R; Camaioni, E., Adenosine deaminase: Functional implications and different classes of inhibitors. *Med. Res. Rev.* 2001, *21* (2), 105-128.

[10]   Silva, RG; Nunes, JES; Canduri, F; Borges, JC; Gava, LM; Moreno, FB; Basso, LA; Santos, DS. Purine nucleoside phosphorylase: a potential target for the development of drugs to treat T-cell- and apicomplexan parasite-mediated diseases. *Curr. Drug Targets*, 2007, *8* (3), 413-422.

[11]   Yuan, G; Bin, JC; McKay, DJ; Snyder, FF. Cloning and characterization of human guanine deaminase. Purification and partial amino acid sequence of the mouse protein. *J. Biol. Chem.* 1999, *274* (12), 8175-8180.

[12]   Battelli, MG; Bolognesi, A; Polito, L. Pathophysiology of circulating xanthine oxidoreductase: New emerging roles for a multi-tasking enzyme. *Biochim. Biophys. Acta (BBA) - Molecular Basis of Disease*, 2014, *1842* (9), 1502-1517.

[13]   Kratzer, JT; Lanaspa, MA; Murphy, MN; Cicerchi, C; Graves, CL; Tipton, PA; Ortlund, EA; Johnson, RJ; Gaucher, EA. Evolutionary history and metabolic insights of ancient mammalian uricases. *Proc. Natl. Acad. Sci. U. S. A.* 2014, *111* (10), 3763-3768.

[14]   Rask-Andersen, M; Masuram, S; Schiöth, HB. The Druggable Genome: Evaluation of drug targets in clinical trials suggests major shifts in molecular class and indication. *Ann. Rev. Pharmacol. Toxicol.* 2014, *54*, 9-26.

[15]   Maurice, DH; Ke, H; Ahmad, F; Wang, Y; Chung, J; Manganiello, VC. Advances in targeting cyclic nucleotide phosphodiesterases. *Nat. Rev. Drug Discov.* 2014, *13* (4), 290-314.

[16]   Manning, BD. Challenges and opportunities in defining the essential cancer kinome. *Sci. Signal.* 2009, *2* (63), pe15.

[17]   Manning, G; Whyte, DB; Martinez, R; Hunter, T; Sudarsanam, S. The Protein Kinase Complement of the Human Genome. *Science*, 2002, *298* (5600), 1912-1916, 1933-1934.

[18]   Cohen, P; Alessi, DR. Kinase drug discovery - What's next in the field? *ACS Chem. Biol.* 2013, *8* (1), 96-104.

[19]   Fabbro, D. 25 years of small molecular weight kinase inhibitors: potentials and limitations. *Mol. Pharmacol.* 2015, *87* (5), 766-775.

[20]   Canavese, M; Santo, L; Raje, N. Cyclin dependent kinases in cancer: potential for therapeutic intervention. *Cancer Biol. Ther.* 2012, *13* (7), 451-457.

[21]   Gallorini, M; Cataldi, A; di Giacomo, V. Cyclin-dependent kinase modulators and cancer therapy. *BioDrugs* 2012, *26* (6), 377-391.

[22]   Stone, A; Sutherland, RL; Musgrove, EA. Inhibitors of cell cycle kinases: recent advances and future prospects as cancer therapeutics. *Crit. Rev. Oncog.* 2012, *17* (2), 175-198.

[23]   Tian, Y; Wan, H; Tan, G. Cell cycle-related kinase in carcinogenesis (review). *Oncol. Lett.* 2012, *4* (4), 601-606.

[24] Jorda, R; Paruch, K; Krystof, V. Cyclin-dependent kinase inhibitors inspired by roscovitine: purine bioisosteres. *Curr. Pharm. Des.* 2012, *18* (20), 2974-2980.

[25] Bettayeb, K; Sallam, H; Ferandin, Y; Popowycz, F; Fournet, G; Hassan, M; Echalier, A; Bernard, P; Endicott, J; Joseph, B; Meijer, L. N-&-N, a new class of cell death-inducing kinase inhibitors derived from the purine roscovitine. *Mol. Cancer Ther.* 2008, *7* (9), 2713-2724.

[26] Popowycz, F; Fournet, G; Schneider, C; Bettayeb, K; Ferandin, Y; Lamigeon, C; Tirado, OM; Mateo-Lozano, S; Notario, V; Colas, P; Bernard, P; Meijer, L; Joseph, B. Pyrazolo[1,5-*a*]-1,3,5-triazine as a purine bioisostere: Access to potent cyclin-dependent kinase inhibitor (*R*)-roscovitine analogue. *J. Med. Chem.* 2009, *52* (3), 655-663.

[27] Jorda, R; Havlicek, L; McNae, IW; Walkinshaw, MD; Voller, J; Sturc, A; Navratilova, J; Kuzma, M; Mistrik, M; Bartek, J; Strnad, M; Krystof, V. Pyrazolo[4,3-*d*]pyrimidine bioisostere of roscovitine: Evaluation of a novel selective inhibitor of cyclin-dependent kinases with antiproliferative activity. *J. Med. Chem.* 2011, *54* (8), 2980-2993.

[28] Montenarh, M., Cellular regulators of protein kinase CK2. *Cell Tissue Res.* 2010, *342* (2), 139-146.

[29] Hanif, IM; Hanif, IM; Shazib, MA; Ahmad, KA; Pervaiz, S. Casein Kinase II: An attractive target for anti-cancer drug design. *Int. J. Biochem. Cell Biol.* 2010, *42* (10), 1602-1605.

[30] Nie, Z; Perretta, C; Erickson, P; Margosiak, S; Almassy, R; Lu, J; Averill, A; Yager, K. M; Chu, S. Structure-based design, synthesis, and study of pyrazolo[1,5-*a*][1,3,5]triazine derivatives as potent inhibitors of protein kinase CK2. *Bioorg. Med. Chem. Lett.* 2007, *17* (15), 4191-4195.

[31] Nie, Z; Perretta, C; Erickson, P; Margosiak, S; Lu, J; Averill, A; Almassy, R; Chu, S. Structure-based design and synthesis of novel macrocyclic pyrazolo[1,5-*a*][1,3,5]triazine compounds as potent inhibitors of protein kinase CK2 and their anticancer activities. *Bioorg. Med. Chem. Lett.* 2008, *18* (2), 619-623.

[32] Keen, N; Taylor, S. Aurora-kinase inhibitors as anticancer agents. *Nat. Rev. Cancer* 2004, *4* (12), 927-936.

[33] Matthews, N; Visintin, C; Hartzoulakis, B; Jarvis, A; Selwood, DL. Aurora A and B kinases as targets for cancer: will they be selective for tumors? *Expert Rev. Anticancer Ther.* 2006, *6* (1), 109-120.

[34] Harrington, EA; Bebbington, D; Moore, J; Rasmussen, RK; Ajose-Adeogun, AO; Nakayama, T; Graham, JA; Demur, C; Hercend, T; Diu-Hercend, A; Su, M; Golec, JMC; Miller, KM. VX-680, a potent and selective small-molecule inhibitor of the Aurora kinases, suppresses tumor growth in vivo. *Nat. Med.* 2004, *10* (3), 262-267.

[35] Fancelli, D; Berta, D; Bindi, S; Cameron, A; Cappella, P; Carpinelli, P; Catana, C; Forte, B; Giordano, P; Giorgini, ML; Mantegani, S; Marsiglio, A; Meroni, M; Moll, J; Pittala, V; Roletto, F; Severino, D; Soncini, C; Storici, P; Tonani, R; Varasi, M; Vulpetti, A; Vianello, P. Potent and selective Aurora inhibitors identified by the expansion of a novel scaffold for protein kinase inhibition. *J. Med. Chem.* 2005, *48* (8), 3080-3084.

[36] Soncini, C; Carpinelli, P; Gianellini, L; Fancelli, D; Vianello, P; Rusconi, L; Storici, P; Zugnoni, P; Pesenti, E; Croci, V; Ceruti, R; Giorgini, ML; Cappella, P; Ballinari, D;

Sola, F; Varasi, M; Bravo, R; Moll, J. PHA-680632, a novel Aurora kinase inhibitor with potent antitumoral activity. *Clin. Cancer Res.* 2006, *12* (13), 4080-4089.

[37] Bavetsias, V; Sun, C; Bouloc, N; Reynisson, J; Workman, P; Linardopoulos, S; McDonald, E. Hit generation and exploration: Imidazo[4,5-*b*]pyridine derivatives as inhibitors of Aurora kinases. *Bioorg. Med. Chem. Lett.* 2007, *17* (23), 6567-6571.

[38] Bavetsias, V; Large, JM; Sun, C; Bouloc, N; Kosmopoulou, M; Matteucci, M; Wilsher, NE; Martins, V; Reynisson, J; Atrash, B; Faisal, A; Urban, F; Valenti, M; Brandon, AdH; Box, G; Raynaud, FI; Workman, P; Eccles, SA; Bayliss, R; Blagg, J; Linardopoulos, S; McDonald, E. Imidazo[4,5-*b*]pyridine derivatives as inhibitors of Aurora kinases: Lead optimization studies toward the identification of an orally bioavailable preclinical development candidate. *J. Med. Chem.* 2010, *53* (14), 5213-5228.

[39] Atrash, B; Faisal, A; Moore, AS; Kosmopoulou, M; Brown, N; Sheldrake, PW; Bush, K; Henley, A; Box, G; Valenti, M; Brandon, AdH; Raynaud, FI; Workman, P; Eccles, SA; Bayliss, R; Linardopoulos, S; Blagg, J. Optimization of imidazo[4,5-*b*]pyridine-based kinase inhibitors: Identification of a dual FLT3/Aurora kinase inhibitor as an orally bioavailable preclinical development candidate for the treatment of acute myeloid leukemia. *J. Med. Chem.* 2012, *55* (20), 8721-8734.

[40] Bavetsias, V; Faisal, A; Crumpler, S; Brown, N; Kosmopoulou, M; Joshi, A; Atrash, B; Perez-Fuertes, Y; Schmitt, JA; Boxall, KJ; Burke, R; Sun, C; Avery, S; Bush, K; Henley, A; Raynaud, FI; Workman, P; Bayliss, R; Linardopoulos, S; Blagg, J. Aurora isoform selectivity: Design and synthesis of imidazo[4,5-*b*]pyridine derivatives as highly selective inhibitors of Aurora A kinase in cells. *J. Med. Chem.* 2013, *56* (22), 9122-9135.

[41] Mohamed, AJ; Yu, L; Backesjo, CM; Vargas, L; Faryal, R; Aints, A; Christensson, B; Berglof, A; Vihinen, M; Nore, BF; Smith, CIE. Bruton's tyrosine kinase (Btk): function, regulation, and transformation with special emphasis on the PH domain. *Immunol. Rev.* 2009, *228* (1), 58-73.

[42] Dinh, M; Grunberger, D; Ho, H; Tsing, SY; Shaw, D; Lee, S; Barnett, J; Hill, RJ; Swinney, D. C; Bradshaw, JM. Activation mechanism and steady state kinetics of Bruton's tyrosine kinase. *J. Biol. Chem.* 2007, *282* (12), 8768-8776.

[43] Jongstra-Bilen, J; Puig, CA; Hasija, M; Xiao, H; Smith, CIE; Cybulsky, MI. Dual functions of Bruton's tyrosine kinase and Tec kinase during Fcγ receptor-induced signaling and phagocytosis. *J. Immunol.* 2008, *181* (1), 288-298.

[44] Hendriks, RW. Drug discovery: New BTK inhibitor holds promise. *Nat. Chem. Biol.* 2011, *7* (1), 4-5.

[45] Xu, D; Kim, Y; Postelnek, J; Vu, M. D; Hu, DQ; Liao, C; Bradshaw, M; Hsu, J; Zhang, J; Pashine, A; Srinivasan, D; Woods, J; Levin, A; O'Mahony, A; Owens, TD; Lou, Y; Hill, RJ; Narula, S; DeMartino, J; Fine, JS. RN486, a selective Bruton's tyrosine kinase inhibitor, abrogates immune hypersensitivity responses and arthritis in rodents. *J. Pharmacol. Exp. Ther.* 2012, *341* (1), 90-103.

[46] Sheridan, C. Companies in rapid pursuit of BTK immunokinase. *Nat. Biotechnol.* 2012, *30* (3), 199-200.

[47] Lou, Y; Owens, TD; Kuglstatter, A; Kondru, RK; Goldstein, DM. Bruton's tyrosine kinase inhibitors: Approaches to potent and selective inhibition, preclinical and clinical

evaluation for inflammatory diseases and B cell malignancies. *J. Med. Chem.* 2012, *55* (10), 4539-4550.

[48] Cameron, F; Sanford, M. Ibrutinib: First global approval. *Drugs*, 2014, *74* (2), 263-271.

[49] Zhao, X; Huang, W; Wang, Y; Xin, M; Jin, Q; Cai, J; Tang, F; Zhao, Y; Xiang, H. Discovery of novel Bruton's tyrosine kinase (BTK) inhibitors bearing a pyrrolo[2,3-*d*]pyrimidine scaffold. *Bioorg. Med. Chem. Lett.* 2015, *23* (4), 891-901.

[50] Thompson, JE. JAK protein kinase inhibitors. *Drug News Perspect.* 2005, *18* (5), 305-310.

[51] Plosker, GL. Ruxolitinib: A review of its use in patients with myelofibrosis. *Drugs*, 2015, *75* (3), 297-308.

[52] Terry, RL; Flechner, SM; Puisis, JW; Miller, SD; Getts, DR. Efficacy and safety of tofacitinib. *J. Symptoms Signs*, 2013, *2* (6), 485-495.

[53] https://clinicaltrials.gov/ct2/show/NCT01251965

[54] https://clinicaltrials.gov/ct2/show/NCT01423604

[55] https://clinicaltrials.gov/ct2/show/NCT01562873

[56] https://clinicaltrials.gov/ct2/show/NCT01877005

[57] https://clinicaltrials.gov/ct2/show/NCT02038036

[58] https://clinicaltrials.gov/ct2/show/NCT01932372

[59] https://clinicaltrials.gov/ct2/show/NCT02312882

[60] https://clinicaltrials.gov/ct2/show/NCT01711359

[61] Mahajan, K; Mahajan, NP. ACK1 tyrosine kinase: Targeted inhibition to block cancer cell proliferation. *Cancer Lett.* 2013, *338* (2), 185-192.

[62] Jiao, X; Kopecky, DJ; Liu, J; Liu, J; Jaen, JC; Cardozo, MG; Sharma, R; Walker, N; Wesche, H; Li, S; Farrelly, E; Xiao, SH; Wang, Z; Kayser, F. Synthesis and optimization of substituted furo[2,3-*d*]-pyrimidin-4-amines and 7*H*-pyrrolo[2,3-*d*]pyrimidin-4-amines as ACK1 inhibitors. *Bioorg. Med. Chem. Lett.* 2012, *22* (19), 6212-6217.

[63] Ingley, E. Src family kinases: Regulation of their activities, levels and identification of new pathways. *Biochim. Biophys. Acta, Proteins Proteomics*, 2008, *1784* (1), 56-65.

[64] Sen, B; Johnson, FM. Regulation of Src family kinases in human cancers. *J. Signal Transduction*, 2011, 865819.

[65] Cao, X; You, QD; Li, ZY; Wang, XJ; Lu, XY; Liu, XR; Xu, D; Liu, B. Recent progress of Src family kinase inhibitors as anticancer agents. *Mini-Rev. Med. Chem.* 2008, *8* (10), 1053-1063.

[66] Hanke, JH; Gardner, JP; Dow, RL; Changelian, PS; Brissette, WH; Weringer, EJ; Pollok, BA; Connelly, PA. Discovery of a novel, potent, and Src family-selective tyrosine kinase inhibitor. Study of Lck- and FynT-dependent T cell activation. *J. Biol. Chem.* 1996, *271* (2), 695-701.

[67] Schenone, S; Brullo, C; Musumeci, F; Biava, M; Falchi, F; Botta, M. Fyn kinase in brain diseases and cancer: the search for inhibitors. *Curr. Med. Chem.*2011, *18* (19), 2921-2942.

[68] Missbach, M; Jeschke, M; Feyen, J; Muller, K; Glatt, M; Green, J; Susa, M. A novel inhibitor of the tyrosine kinase Src suppresses phosphorylation of its major cellular substrates and reduces bone resorption *in vitro* and in rodent models *in vivo*. *Bone*, 1999, *24* (5), 437-449.

[69] Missbach, M; Altmann, E; Widler, L; Susa, M; Buchdunger, E; Mett, H; Meyer, T; Green, J., Substituted 5,7-diphenylpyrrolo[2,3-*d*]pyrimidines: potent inhibitors of the tyrosine kinase c-Src. *Bioorg. Med. Chem. Lett.* 2000, *10* (9), 945-949.

[70] Šuša, M; Luong-Nguyen, NH; Crespo, J; Maier, R; Missbach, M; McMaster, G. Active recombinant human Tyrosine kinase c-Yes: Expression in baculovirus system, purification, comparison to c-Src, and inhibition by a c-Src inhibitor. *Protein Expr. Purif.* 2000, *19* (1), 99-106.

[71] Recchia, I; Rucci, N; Festuccia, C; Bologna, M; MacKay, AR; Migliaccio, S; Longo, M; Susa, M; Fabbro, D; Teti, A. Pyrrolopyrimidine c-Src inhibitors reduce growth, adhesion, motility and invasion of prostate cancer cells in vitro. *Eur. J. Cancer,* 2003, *39* (13), 1927-1935.

[72] Wilson, MB; Schreiner, SJ; Choi, HJ; Kamens, J; Smithgall, TE. Selective pyrrolo-pyrimidine inhibitors reveal a necessary role for Src family kinases in Bcr-Abl signal transduction and oncogenesis. *Oncogene,* 2002, *21* (53), 8075-8088.

[73] Labbe, C; Ross, OA. Association studies of sporadic Parkinson's disease in the genomic era. *Curr. Genomics,* 2014, *15* (1), 2-10.

[74] Lubbe, S; Morris, HR. Recent advances in Parkinson's disease genetics. *J. Neurol.* 2014, *261* (2), 259-266.

[75] Healy, DG; Falchi, M; O'Sullivan, SS; Bonifati, V; Durr, A; Bressman, S; Brice, A; Aasly, J; Zabetian, CP; Goldwurm, S; Ferreira, JJ; Tolosa, E; Kay, DM; Klein, C; Williams, DR; Marras, C; Lang, AE; Wszolek, ZK; Berciano, J; Schapira, AHV; Lynch, T; Bhatia, KP; Gasser, T; Lees, AJ; Wood, NW. Phenotype, genotype, and worldwide genetic penetrance of LRRK2-associated Parkinson's disease: a case-control study. *Lancet Neurol.* 2008, *7* (7), 583-590.

[76] Henderson, J. L; Kormos, B. L; Hayward, M. M; Coffman, K. J; Jasti, J; Kurumbail, R. G; Wager, T. T; Verhoest, P. R; Noell, G. S; Chen, Y; Needle, E; Berger, Z; Steyn, S. J; Houle, C; Hirst, W. D; Galatsis, P., Discovery and preclinical profiling of 3-[4-(morpholin-4-yl)-7H-pyrrolo[2,3-*d*]pyrimidin-5-yl]benzonitrile (PF-06447475),   a highly potent, selective, brain penetrant, and *in vivo* active LRRK2 kinase inhibitor. *J. Med. Chem.* 2015, *58* (1), 419-432.

[77] Hatcher, JM; Zhang, J; Choi, HG; Ito, G; Alessi, DR; Gray, NS. Discovery of a pyrrolopyrimidine (JH-II-127), a highly potent, selective, and brain penetrant LRRK2 inhibitor. *ACS Med. Chem. Lett.* 2015, *6* (5), 584-589.

[78] Francis, SH; Blount, MA; Corbin, JD. Mammalian cyclic nucleotide phosphodiesterases: molecular mechanisms and physiological functions. *Physiol. Rev.* 2011, *91* (2), 651-690.

[79] Amer, MS. Cyclic nucleotides as targets for drug design. *Adv. Drug Res.* 1977, *12*, 1-38.

[80] Dent, G; Rabe, K. F., Effects of theophylline and non-selective xanthine derivatives on PDE isoenzymes and cellular function. *Phosphodiesterase Inhibitors*, Dent, C. S; Rabe, K. F., Eds. Academic Press: San Diego, 1996; pp 41-64.

[81] Gibson, A. Phosphodiesterase 5 inhibitors and nitrergic transmission-from zaprinast to sildenafil. *Eur. J. Pharmacol.* 2001, *411* (1-2), 1-10.

[82] Rotella, DP. Phosphodiesterase 5 inhibitors: current status and potential applications. *Nat. Rev. Drug Discov.* 2002, *1* (9), 674-682.

[83]   Kim, DK; Lee, N; Lee, JY; Ryu, DH; Kim, JS; Lee, SH; Choi, JY; Chang, K; Kim, YW; Im, GJ; Choi, WS; Kim, TK; Ryu, JH; Kim, NH; Lee, K. Synthesis and phosphodiesterase 5 inhibitory activity of novel phenyl ring modified sildenafil analogues. *Bioorg. Med. Chem.* 2001, *9* (6), 1609-1616.

[84]   Kim, DK; Lee, JY; Lee, N; Ryu, DH; Kim, JS; Lee, S; Choi, JY; Ryu, JH; Kim, NH; Im, GJ; Choi, WS; Kim, TK. Synthesis and phosphodiesterase inhibitory activity of new sildenafil analogs containing a carboxylic acid group in the 5'-sulfonamide moiety of the phenyl ring. *Bioorg. Med. Chem.* 2001, *9* (11), 3013-3021.

[85]   Kim, DK; Ryu, DH; Lee, N; Lee, JY; Kim, JS; Lee, S; Choi, JY; Ryu, J. H; Kim, NH; Im, GJ; Choi, WS; Kim, TK. Synthesis and phosphodiesterase 5 inhibitory activity of new 5-phenyl-1,6-dihydro-7H-pyrazolo[4,3-*d*]pyrimidin-7-one derivatives containing an N-acylamido group on a phenyl ring. *Bioorg. Med. Chem.* 2001, *9* (7), 1895-1899.

[86]   Haning, H; Niewoehner, U; Schenke, T; Lampe, T; Hillisch, A; Bischoff, E. Comparison of different heterocyclic scaffolds as substrate analog PDE5 inhibitors. *Bioorg. Med. Chem. Lett.* 2005, *15* (17), 3900-3907.

[87]   Haning, H; Niewohner, U; Schenke, T; Es-Sayed, M; Schmidt, G; Lampe, T; Bischoff, E. Imidazo[5,1-*f*]triazin-4(3H)-ones, a new class of potent PDE5 inhibitors. *Bioorg. Med. Chem. Lett.* 2002, *12* (6), 865-868.

[88]   Sawant, SD; Lakshma Reddy, G; Dar, MI; Srinivas, M; Gupta, G; Sahu, PK; Mahajan, P; Nargotra, A; Singh, S; Sharma, SC; Tikoo, M; Singh, G; Vishwakarma, RA; Syed, SH. Discovery of novel pyrazolopyrimidinone analogs as potent inhibitors of phosphodiesterase type-5. *Bioorg. Med. Chem.* 2015, *23* (9), 2121-2128.

[89]   Fisher, DA; Smith, JF; Pillar, JS; Denis, SHS; Cheng, JB. Isolation and characterization of PDE9A, a novel human cGMP-specific phosphodiesterase. *J. Biol. Chem.* 1998, *273* (25), 15559-15564.

[90]   Wang, P; Wu, P; Egan, RW; Billah, MM. Identification and characterization of a new human type 9 cGMP-specific phosphodiesterase splice variant (PDE9A5). Differential tissue distribution and subcellular localization of PDE9A variants. *Gene,* 2003, *314,* 15-27.

[91]   Wunder, F; Tersteegen, A; Rebmann, A; Erb, C; Fahrig, T; Hendrix, M. Characterization of the first potent and selective PDE9 inhibitor using a cGMP reporter cell line. *Mol. Pharmacol.* 2005, *68* (6), 1775-1781.

[92]   DeNinno, MP; Andrews, M; Bell, AS; Chen, Y; Eller-Zarbo, C; Eshelby, N; Etienne, JB; Moore, DE; Palmer, MJ; Visser, MS; Yu, LJ; Zavadoski, WJ; Gibbs, EM. The discovery of potent, selective, and orally bioavailable PDE9 inhibitors as potential hypoglycemic agents. *Bioorg. Med. Chem. Lett.* 2009, *19* (9), 2537-2541.

[93]   Wager, TT; Hou, X; Verhoest, PR; Villalobos, A. Moving beyond rules: The development of a Central Nervous System Multiparameter Optimization (CNS MPO) approach to enable alignment of druglike properties. *ACS Chem. Neurosci.* 2010, *1* (6), 435-449.

[94]   Hutson, PH; Finger, EN; Magliaro, BC; Smith, SM; Converso, A; Sanderson, PE; Mullins, D; Hyde, LA; Eschle, BK; Turnbull, Z; Sloan, H; Guzzi, M; Zhang, X; Wang, A; Rindgen, D; Mazzola, R; Vivian, J. A; Eddins, D; Uslaner, J. M; Bednar, R; Gambone, C; Le-Mair, W; Marino, MJ; Sachs, N; Xu, G; Parmentier-Batteur, S. The selective phosphodiesterase 9 (PDE9) inhibitor PF-04447943 (6-[((3S,4S)-4-methyl-1-(pyrimidin-2-ylmethyl)pyrrolidin-3-yl]-1-(tetrahydro-2H-pyran-4-yl)-1,5-dihydro-4H-

pyrazolo[3,4-*d*]pyrimidin-4-one) enhances synaptic plasticity and cognitive function in rodents. *Neuropharmacology*, 2011, *61* (4), 665-676.

[95] Verhoest, PR; Proulx-Lafrance, C; Corman, M; Chenard, L; Helal, CJ; Hou, X; Kleiman, R; Liu, S; Marr, E; Menniti, FS; Schmidt, CJ; Vanase-Frawley, M; Schmidt, AW; Williams, RD; Nelson, FR; Fonseca, KR; Liras, S. Identification of a brain penetrant PDE9A inhibitor utilizing prospective design and chemical enablement as a rapid lead optimization strategy. *J. Med. Chem.* 2009, *52* (24), 7946-7949.

[96] Fisher, DA; Smith, JF; Pillar, JS; St. Denis, SH; Cheng, JB. Isolation and characterization of PDE8A, a novel human cAMP-specific phosphodiesterase. *Biochem. Biophys. Res. Commun.* 1998, *246* (3), 570-577.

[97] Hayashi, M; Matsushima, K; Ohashi, H; Tsunoda, H; Murase, S; Kawarada, Y; Tanaka, T. Molecular cloning and characterization of human PDE8B, a novel thyroid-specific isoenzyme of 3',5'-cyclic nucleotide phosphodiesterase. *Biochem. Biophys. Res. Commun.* 1998, *250* (3), 751-756.

[98] Vang, AG; Ben-Sasson, SZ; Dong, H; Kream, B; DeNinno, MP; Claffey, MM; Housley, W; Clark, RB; Epstein, PM; Brocke, S. PDE8 regulates rapid Teff cell adhesion and proliferation independent of ICER. *PLoS One*, 2010, *5* (8) e12011.

[99] Shimizu-Albergine, M; Tsai, LC. L; Patrucco, E; Beavo, JA. cAMP-specific phosphodiesterases 8A and 8B, essential regulators of Leydig cell steroidogenesis. *Mol. Pharmacol.* 2012, *81* (4), 556-566.

[100] DeNinno, MP; Wright, SW; Etienne, JB; Olson, TV; Rocke, BN; Corbett, JW; Kung, DW; DiRico, KJ; Andrews, KM; Millham, ML; Parker, JC; Esler, W; van Volkenburg, M; Boyer, DD; Houseknecht, KL; Doran, SD. Discovery of triazolopyrimidine-based PDE8B inhibitors: Exceptionally ligand-efficient and lipophilic ligand-efficient compounds for the treatment of diabetes. *Bioorg. Med. Chem. Lett.* 2012, *22* (17), 5721-5726.

[101] Zhang, C; Yu, Y; Ruan, L; Wang, C; Pan, J; Klabnik, J; Lueptow, L; Zhang, HT; O'Donnell, JM; Xu, Y. The roles of phosphodiesterase 2 in the central nervous and peripheral systems. *Curr. Pharm. Des.* 2015, *21* (3), 274-290.

[102] Bessodes, M; Bastian, G; Abushanab, E; Panzica, RP; Berman, SF; Marcaccio, EJ., Jr; Chen, SF; Stoeckler, JD; Parks, RE. Jr. Effect of chirality in erythro-9-(2-hydroxy-3-nonyl)adenine (EHNA) on adenosine deaminase inhibition. *Biochem. Pharmacol.* 1982, *31* (5), 879-882.

[103] Méry, PF; Pavoine, C; Pecker, F; Fischmeister, R. EHNA as an inhibitor of PDE2: A pharmacological and biochemical study in cardiac myocytes. *Phosphodiesterase Inhibitors*, Dent, C. S; Rabe, K. F., Eds. Academic Press: San Diego, 1996; pp 81-88.

[104] Boess, FG; Hendrix, M; van der Staay, FJ; Erb, C; Schreiber, R; van Staveren, W; de Vente, J; Prickaerts, J; Blokland, A; Koenig, G. Inhibition of phosphodiesterase 2 increases neuronal cGMP, synaptic plasticity and memory performance. *Neuropharmacology*, 2004, *47* (7), 1081-1092.

[105] Domek-Lopacinska, K; Strosznajder, JB. The effect of selective inhibition of cyclic GMP hydrolyzing phosphodiesterases 2 and 5 on learning and memory processes and nitric oxide synthase activity in brain during aging. *Brain Res.* 2008, *1216*, 68-77.

[106] Masood, A; Huang, Y; Hajjhussein, H; Xiao, L; Li, H; Wang, W; Hamza, A; Zhan, CG; O'Donnell, JM. Anxiolytic effects of phosphodiesterase-2 inhibitors associated with increased cGMP signaling. *J. Pharmacol. Exp. Ther.* 2009, *331* (2), 690-699.

[107] Xu, Y; Pan, J; Chen, L; Zhang, C; Sun, J; Li, J; Nguyen, L; Nair, N; Zhang, H; O'Donnell, JM. Phosphodiesterase-2 inhibitor reverses corticosterone-induced neurotoxicity and related behavioural changes via cGMP/PKG dependent pathway. *Int. J. Neuropsychopharmacol.* 2013, *16* (4), 835-847.

[108] Helal, CJ; Chappie, TA; Humphrey, JM. Preparation of pyrazolopyrimidine derivatives for use as PDE2 and/or CYP3A4 inhibitors. Patent 2WO 2012168817.

[109] Helal, CJ; Chappie, TA; Humphrey, JM; Verhoest, PR; Yang, E. Preparation of imidazo[5,1-*f*][1,2,4]triazines for the treatment of neurological disorders. Patent 2US 20120214791.

[110] Helal, CJ; Chappie, T; Humphrey, J; Verhoest, P; Yang, E; Arnold, E; Bundesmann, M; Hou, X; Kormos, B; Mente, S; Kleiman, R; Pandit, J; Schmidt, C. Identification of a brain penetrant, highly selective phosphodiesterase 2A inhibitor clinical candidate for treating cognitive impairment: In vivo efficacy and human pharmacokinetic data. *Abstracts of Papers, 248th ACS National Meeting & Exposition, San Francisco, CA, United States, August 10-14,* 2014, MEDI-275.

[111] Kurz, LC; Frieden, C. Adenosine deaminase converts purine riboside into an analog of a reactive intermediate: a carbon-13 NMR and kinetic study. *Biochemistry* 1987, *26* (25), 8450-7.

[112] Aiuti, A. Advances in gene therapy for ADA-deficient SCID. *Curr. Opin. Mol. Ther.* 2002, *4* (5), 515-522.

[113] Rafel, M; Cervantes, F; Beltran, JM; Zuazu, F; Nieto, LH; Rayon, C; Talavera, JG; Montserrat, E. Deoxycoformycin in the treatment of patients with hairy cell leukemia: results of a Spanish collaborative study of 80 patients. *Cancer,* 2000, *88* (2), 352-357.

[114] Honma, Y. A novel therapeutic strategy against monocytic leukemia with deoxyadenosine analogs and adenosine deaminase inhibitors. *Leuk. Lymphoma,* 2001, *42* (5), 953-962.

[115] Tofovic, SP; Kusaka, H; Li, P; Jackson, EK. Effects of adenosine deaminase inhibition on blood pressure in old spontaneously hypertensive rats. *Clin. Exp. Hypertens.* 1998, *20* (3), 329-344.

[116] Mandapathil, M; Hilldorfer, B; Szczepanski, MJ; Czystowska, M; Szajnik, M; Ren, J; Lang, S; Jackson, EK; Gorelik, E; Whiteside, TL. Generation and accumulation of immunosuppressive adenosine by human $CD4^+CD25^{high}FOXP3^+$ regulatory T cells. *J. Biol. Chem.* 2010, *285* (10), 7176-7186.

[117] Hosmane, RS. Ring-expanded ("fat") nucleosides as broad-spectrum anticancer and antiviral agents. *Curr. Top. Med. Chem.* 2002, *2* (10), 1093-1109.

[118] Schaeffer, HJ; Schwender, CF. Enzyme inhibitors. 26. Bridging hydrophobic and hydrophilic regions on adenosine deaminase with some 9-(2-hydroxy-3-alkyl)adenines. *J. Med. Chem.* 1974, *17* (1), 6-8.

[119] Kurz, LC; Weitkamp, E; Frieden, C. Adenosine deaminase: viscosity studies and the mechanism of binding of substrate and of ground- and transition-state analog inhibitors. *Biochemistry,* 1987, *26* (11), 3027-3032.

[120] Pragnacharyulu, PVP; Lu, PJ; Abushanab, E. Adenosine deaminase inhibitors. Synthesis and biological evaluation of chain modified analogs of (+)-EHNA. *Bioorg. Med. Chem. Lett.* 1996, *6* (20), 2417-2420.

[121] McConnell, WR; El Dareer, SM; Hill, DL. Metabolism and disposition of *erythro*-9-(2-hydroxy-3-nonyl)[^{14}C]adenine in the rhesus monkey. *Drug Metab. Dispos.* 1980, *8* (1), 5-7.

[122] Da Settimo, F; Primofiore, G; La Motta, C; Taliani, S; Simorini, F; Marini, AM; Mugnaini, L; Lavecchia, A; Novellino, E; Tuscano, D; Martini, C. Novel, highly potent adenosine deaminase inhibitors containing the pyrazolo[3,4-*d*]pyrimidine ring system. Synthesis, structure-activity relationships, and molecular modeling studies. *J. Med. Chem.* 2005, *48* (16), 5162-5174.

[123] Antonioli, L; Fornai, M; Colucci, R; Ghisu, N; Da Settimo, F; Natale, G; Kastsiuchenka, O; Duranti, E; Virdis, A; Vassalle, C; La Motta, C; Mugnaini, L; Breschi, MC; Blandizzi, C; Del Tacca, M. Inhibition of adenosine deaminase attenuates inflammation in experimental colitis. *J. Pharmacol. Exp. Ther.* 2007, *322* (2), 435-442.

[124] La Motta, C; Sartini, S; Mugnaini, L; Salerno, S; Simorini, F; Taliani, S; Marini, AM; Da Settimo, F; Lavecchia, A; Novellino, E; Antonioli, L; Fornai, M; Blandizzi, C; Del Tacca, M. Exploiting the pyrazolo[3,4-*d*]pyrimidin-4-one ring system as a useful template to obtain potent adenosine deaminase inhibitors. *J. Med. Chem.* 2009, *52* (6), 1681-1692.

[125] Milton, JM; Konuk, M; Brown, EG. *Lepista nebularis* — Producer of nebularine. *Mycologist*, 1992, *6* (1), 44-45.

[126] Shewach, DS; Krawczyk, SH; Acevedo, OL; Townsend, LB. Inhibition of adenosine deaminase by azapurine ribonucleosides. *Biochem. Pharmacol.* 1992, *44* (9), 1697-700.

[127] Bzowska, A; Kulikowska, E; Shugar, D. Purine nucleoside phosphorylases: properties, functions, and clinical aspects. *Pharmacol. Therapeut.* 2000, *88* (3), 349-425.

[128] Korycka, A; Blonski, JZ; Robak, T. Forodesine (BCX-1777, immucillin H) - a new purine nucleoside analogue: mechanism of action and potential clinical application. *Mini-Rev. Med. Chem.* 2007, *7* (9), 976-983.

[129] Kicska, GA; Long, L; Horig, H; Fairchild, C; Tyler, PC; Furneaux, RH; Schramm, VL; Kaufman, HL. Immucillin H, a powerful transition-state analog inhibitor of purine nucleoside phosphorylase, selectively inhibits human T lymphocytes. *Proc. Natl. Acad. Sci. U. S. A.* 2001, *98* (8), 4593-4598.

[130] Robak, P; Robak, T. Older and new purine nucleoside analogs for patients with acute leukaemias. *Cancer Treat. Rev.* 2013, *39* (8), 851-861.

[131] Gandhi, V; Kilpatrick, JM; Plunkett, W; Ayres, M; Harman, L; Du, M; Bantia, S; Davisson, J; Wierda, WG; Faderl, S; Kantarjian, H; Thomas, D. A proof-of-principle pharmacokinetic, pharmacodynamic, and clinical study with purine nucleoside phosphorylase inhibitor immucillin-H (BCX-1777, forodesine). *Blood*, 2005, *106* (13), 4253-4260.

[132] Bantia, S; Parker, C; Upshaw, R; Cunningham, A; Kotian, P; Kilpatrick, JM; Morris, P; Chand, P; Babu, YS. Potent orally bioavailable purine nucleoside phosphorylase inhibitor BCX-4208 induces apoptosis in B- and T-lymphocytes-A novel treatment approach for autoimmune diseases, organ transplantation and hematologic malignancies. *Int. Immunopharmacol.* 2010, *10* (7), 784-790.

[133] Mason, JM; Murkin, AS; Li, L; Schramm, VL; Gainsford, GJ; Skelton, BW. A β-fluoroamine inhibitor of purine nucleoside phosphorylase. *J. Med. Chem.* 2008, *51* (18), 5880-5884.

[134] Halazy, S; Ehrhard, A; Danzin, C. 9-(Difluorophosphonoalkyl)guanines as a new class of multisubstrate analog inhibitors of purine nucleoside phosphorylase. *J. Am. Chem. Soc.* 1991, *113* (1), 315-317.

[135] Hikishima, S; Hashimoto, M; Magnowska, L; Bzowska, A; Yokomatsu, T. Synthesis and biological evaluation of 9-deazaguanine derivatives connected by a linker to difluoromethylene phosphonic acid as multi-substrate analogue inhibitors of PNP. *Bioorg. Med. Chem. Lett.* 2007, *17* (15), 4173-4177.

[136] Hikishima, S; Hashimoto, M; Magnowska, L; Bzowska, A; Yokomatsu, T. Structural-based design and synthesis of novel 9-deazaguanine derivatives having a phosphate mimic as multi-substrate analogue inhibitors for mammalian PNPs. *Bioorg. Med. Chem.* 2010, *18* (6), 2275-2284.

[137] Breer, K; Glavaš-Obrovac, L; Suver, M; Hikishima, S; Hashimoto, M; Yokomatsu, T; Wielgus-Kutrowska, B; Magnowska, L; Bzowska, A. 9-Deazaguanine derivatives connected by a linker to difluoromethylene phosphonic acid are slow-binding picomolar inhibitors of trimeric purine nucleoside phosphorylase. *FEBS J.* 2010, *277* (7), 1747-1760.

[138] Glavaš-Obrovac, L; Suver, M; Hikishima, S; Hashimoto, M; Yokomatsu, T; Magnowska, L; Bzowska, A. Antiproliferative activity of purine nucleoside phosphorylase multisubstrate analogue inhibitors containing difluoromethylene phosphonic acid against leukaemia and lymphoma cells. *Chem. Biol. Drug Des.* 2010, *75* (4), 392-399.

[139] Hille, R; Nishino, T. Xanthine oxidase and xanthine dehydrogenase. *FASEB J.* 1995, *9* (11), 995-1003.

[140] Chao, J; Terkeltaub, R., A critical reappraisal of allopurinol dosing, safety, and efficacy for hyperuricemia in gout. *Curr. Rheumatol. Rep.* 2009, *11* (2), 135-140.

[141] Robins, RK; Revankar, GR; O'Brien, DE; Springer, RH; Novinson, T; Albert, A; Senga, K; Miller, JP; Streeter, DG. Purine analog inhibitors of xanthine oxidase - structure activity relationships and proposed binding of the molybdenum cofactor. *J. Heterocycl. Chem.* 1985, *22* (3), 601-634.

[142] Fujii, S; Kawamura, H; Kiyokawa, H; Yamada, S. Preparation of pyrazolotriazines as xanthine oxidase inhibitors. Patent 1EP 269859.

[143] Sato, S; Tatsumi, K; Nishino, T. A novel xanthine dehydrogenase inhibitor (BOF-4272). *Adv. Exp. Med. Biol.* 1991, *309A* (Purine Pyrimidine Metab. Man 7, Pt. A), 135-138.

[144] Okamoto, K. New inhibitor of xanthine oxidase. *Yokohama Igaku* 1994, *45* (1), 47-53.

[145] Okamoto, K; Nishino, T. Mechanism of inhibition of xanthine oxidase with a new tight binding inhibitor. *J. Biol. Chem.* 1995, *270* (14), 7816-7821.

[146] Naito, S; Nishimura, M; Tamao, Y. Evaluation of the pharmacological actions and pharmacokinetics of BOF-4272, a xanthine oxidase inhibitor, in mouse liver. *J. Pharm. Pharmacol.* 2000, *52* (2), 173-179.

[147] Uematsu, T; Nakashima, M. Pharmacokinetic and pharmacodynamic properties of a novel xanthine oxidase inhibitor, BOF-4272, in healthy volunteers. *J. Pharmacol. Exp. Ther.* 1994, *270* (2), 453-459.

[148] Suzuki, H; Suematsu, M; Ishii, H; Kato, S; Miki, H; Mori, M; Ishimura, Y; Nishino, T; Tsuchiya, M. Prostaglandin E1 abrogates early reductive stress and zone-specific

paradoxical oxidative injury in hypoperfused rat liver. *J. Clin. Invest.* 1994, *93* (1), 155-164.

[149] Naito, S; Nishimura, M. Enantioselective uptake of BOF-4272, a xanthine oxidase inhibitor with a chiral sulfoxide, by isolated rat hepatocytes. *Yakugaku Zasshi*, 2001, *121* (12), 989-994.

[150] Naito, S; Nishimura, M. In vitro and in vivo studies on the stereoselective pharmacokinetics and biotransformation of an (*S*)-(-)- and (*R*)-(+)-pyrazolotriazine sulfoxide in the male rat. *Xenobiotica*, 2002, *32* (6), 491-503.

[151] Naito, S; Nishimura, M., Stereoselective pharmacokinetics of BOF-4272 racemate after oral administration to rats and dogs. *Biol. Pharm. Bull.* 2002, *25* (5), 674-677.

[152] Matsugi, M; Hashimoto, K; Inai, M; Fukuda, N; Furuta, T; Minamikawa, Ji; Otsuka, S. Asymmetric synthesis of a xanthine dehydrogenase inhibitor (*S*)-(-)-BOF-4272: Utility of chiral alkoxysulfonium salts. *Tetrahedron: Asymmetry*, 1995, *6* (12), 2991-3000.

[153] Hashimoto, K; Matsugi, M; Fukuda, N; Kurogi, Y. Asymmetric synthesis of xanthine dehydrogenase inhibitor (*S*)-(-)-BOF-4272: mechanism of chiral diaryl sulfoxide formation. *Phosphorus Sulfur Silicon Relat. Elem.* 1997, *120 & 121*, 305-315.

[154] Gupta, S; Rodrigues, LM; Esteves, AP; Oliveira-Campos, AMF; Nascimento, MSJ; Nazareth, N; Cidade, H; Neves, MP; Fernandes, E; Pinto, M; Cerqueira, NMFSA; Bras, N. Synthesis of N-aryl-5-amino-4-cyanopyrazole derivatives as potent xanthine oxidase inhibitors. *Eur. J. Med. Chem.* 2008, *43* (4), 771-780.

[155] Kahn, K; Serfozo, P; Tipton, PA. Identification of the true product of the urate oxidase reaction. *J. Am. Chem. Soc.* 1997, *119* (23), 5435-5442.

[156] Oda, M; Satta, Y; Takenaka, O; Takahata, N. Loss of urate oxidase activity in hominoids and its evolutionary implications. *Mol. Biol. Evol.* 2002, *19* (5), 640-653.

[157] Ames, BN; Cathcart, R; Schwiers, E; Hochstein, P. Uric acid provides an antioxidant defense in humans against oxidant- and radical-caused aging and cancer: a hypothesis. *Proc. Natl. Acad. Sci. U. S. A.* 1981, *78* (11), 6858-6862.

[158] Whiteman, M; Halliwell, B. Protection against peroxynitrite-dependent tyrosine nitration and α1-antiproteinase inactivation by ascorbic acid. A comparison with other biological antioxidants. *Free Radical Res.* 1996, *25* (3), 275-283.

[159] Amaral, AC; Fernandes, L; Galdino, AS; Felipe, MSS; Soares, CMdA; Pereira, M. Therapeutic targets in *Paracoccidioides brasiliensis*: Post-transcriptome perspectives. *GMR, Genet. Mol. Res.* 2005, *4* (2), 430-449.

[160] Felipe, MSS; Andrade, RV; Arraes, FBM; Nicola, AM; Maranhao, AQ; Torres, FAG; Silva-Pereira, I; Pocas-Fonseca, MJ; Campos, EG; Moraes, LMP; Andrade, PA; Tavares, AHFP; Silva, SS; Kyaw, CM; Souza, DP; Pereira, M; Jesuino, RSA; Andrade, EV; Parente, JA; Oliveira, GS; Barbosa, MS; Martins, NF; Fachin, AL; Cardoso, RS; Passos, GAS; Almeida, NF; Walter, MEMT; Soares, CMA; Carvalho, MJA; Brigido, MM. Transcriptional profiles of the human pathogenic fungus *Paracoccidioides brasiliensis* in mycelium and yeast cells. *J. Biol. Chem.* 2005, *280* (26), 24706-24714.

[161] Lee, IR; Yang, L; Sebetso, G; Allen, R; Doan, THN; Blundell, R; Lui, EYL; Morrow, CA; Fraser, JA. Characterization of the complete uric acid degradation pathway in the fungal pathogen *Cryptococcus neoformans*. *PLoS One*, 2013, *8* (5), e64292.

[162] Iwata, H; Yamamoto, I; Gohda, E; Morita, K; Nakamura, M; Sumi, K. Potent competitive uricase inhibitors. 2,8-Diazahypoxanthine and related compounds. *Biochem. Pharmacol.* 1973, *22* (18), 2237-2245.

[163] Colloc'h, N; Prange, T. Functional relevance of the internal hydrophobic cavity of urate oxidase. *FEBS Lett.* 2014, *588* (9), 1715-1719.

[164] Collings, I; Watier, Y; Giffard, M; Dagogo, S; Kahn, R; Bonnete, F; Wright, JP; Fitch, AN; Margiolaki, I. Polymorphism of microcrystalline urate oxidase from *Aspergillus flavus*. *Acta Crystallogr. Sect. D Biol. Crystallogr.* 2010, *66* (5), 539-548.

[165] Oksanen, E; Blakeley, MP; Bonnete, F; Dauvergne, MT; Dauvergne, F; Budayova-Spano, M. Large crystal growth by thermal control allows combined X-ray and neutron crystallographic studies to elucidate the protonation states in *Aspergillus flavus* urate oxidase. *J. Royal Soc. Interface*, 2009, *6* (Suppl. 5), S599-S610.

In: Pharmaceutical Formulation
Editor: Bruce Moore

ISBN: 978-1-63484-082-8
© 2015 Nova Science Publishers, Inc.

Chapter 3

L-DOPA DETERMINATION EMPLOYING AN ELECTROCHEMICAL SENSOR BASED ON CARBON NANOTUBE MODIFIED WITH COBALT PHTHALOCYANINE

Ana Elisa Ferreira de Oliveira[*]
and Arnaldo César Pereira[†]

Universidade Federal de São João del-Rei (UFSJ),
Departamento de Ciências Naturais, São João del-Rei, MG, Brazil

ABSTRACT

A new sensitive voltammetric sensor was developed for electrochemical determination of L-Dopa in pharmaceutical formulations with a glassy carbon electrode (GCE) modified with cobalt phthalocyanine (CoPc) adsorbed on multi-walled carbon nanotubes (MWCN). The electrochemical characterization was performed by Scanning Electron Microscopy (SEM) and Fourier Transform Infrared Spectroscopy (FT-IR). The results have shown that MWCN and CoPc form a composite material without formation of large agglomerates. An estimation of the kinetic parameters α (charge transfer coefficient) and κ (heterogeneous transfer rate constant) was carried out using the Laviron's model resulting in α = 0.54 and κ = 22.55 s^{-1}. These results suggest that the GCE immobilized with CoPc forms a quasi-reversible with high transfer speed response. Thus demonstrating that the sensor is kinetically viable for electrooxidation of CoPc, enabling its use as a catalyst for redox processes of various electroactive species. The optimized conditions of the developed system were: MWCN (2.0 mg.mL^{-1}) and CoPc (2.0 mg.mL^{-1}) in 0.1 mol.L^{-1} pH 7.5 phosphate buffered saline. The operational parameters of electroanalytical DPV and SWV were optimized, and the DPV showed higher sensitivity. Therefore the DPV was chosen for the determination of L-Dopa in the pharmaceutical formulation. An analytical curve was made showing a linear response over the concentration range from 10 to 80 µmol.L^{-1}, with R = 0.999. The *limit* of

---

[*] A. C. Pereira: Email: arnaldocsp@yahoo.com.br
[†] A. E. F. Oliveira: Email: ana_elisa_oliveira@yahoo.com

detection (LOD) and the *limit* of *quantification (LOQ)* obtained was equal to 3.7636 and 12.545 $\mu mol.L^{-1}$, respectively. The validation of the proposed electroanalytical method for the determination of L-Dopa was performed according to ANVISA. The precision and accuracy values obtained by *validate* the *method*, were less than 5% maximum recommended by Resolution No. 899 of ANVISA. Therefore, proposed method for determination of L-Dopa was considered accurate and able to be applied to real samples. The developed sensor applied in real samples presented a good recovery with values between 98.50, 98.64% 99.18%, attesting the accuracy of the procedure.

Keywords: Cobalt phthalocyanine, carbon nanotube, L-Dopa

1. INTRODUCTION

The term Chemically Modified Electrode (CME) was introduced by Murray et al. (Morita et al. 2011) in 1975 to indicate electrodes with chemically active species immobilized on their surfaces in order to pre-establish and control the physical-chemical nature of electrode/solution interface. The deliberate modification of electrode surface being a way to order and control their reactivity and/or selectivity enables the development of electrodes for various purposes and applications (Souza 1997).

The application of a CME is extremely important in situations where the analyte has a slow redox reaction at the electrode surface. Using a CME the possibility of making a faster reaction is increased due the presence of electrochemically active species in which there is a mediation of electron transfer causing the reaction to become faster, thus reducing the activation overpotential of reaction (Souza 1997).

A CME consists of two parts: the electrode base and a layer of the modifier. The preparation of a CME is determined by the analytical characteristics desired of the sensor (Pereira 2003). The choice of material for the electrode base, which the surface will be modified, is a very important aspect of the preparation of a CME. This material should present appropriate electrochemical characteristics and also be suitable for the selected immobilization method. Among conventional materials may be mentioned gold, platinum, mercury in the form of film, carbon fibers, carbon paste, carbon nanotube and glassy carbon (Pereira 2003).

The carbon nanotube (CN) exhibit characteristics such as versatility, low background current, low noise, low cost, wide range of working potential, readily renewable surface and possibility of miniaturization (Dias 2003). CN have the highest mechanical strength among all known materials - do not break or deform when bent or subjected to high pressure. Also noteworthy as the best thermal conductor and may be capable of carrying electricity (Herbst, 2004). Besides allowing an easy incorporation of supports and mediators that increase the variety of applications. An example of a metal complex that can be used for modifying the carbon nanotubes are phthalocyanines.

Phthalocyanines were discovered in 1907 by Braun and Tcherniac, and are a class of organic compounds with intense blue color (Canevari 2008). They consist of a set of rings with four separate units that are joined by nitrogen atoms and has two central hydrogen atoms (Todd et al. 1998). These two hydrogen atoms may be replaced by various metals, such as cobalt (Figure 1).

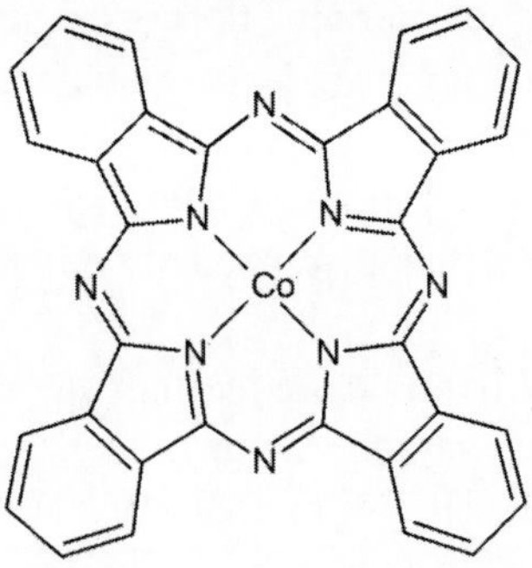

Figure 1. Structural formula of cobalt phthalocyanine.

The cobalt phthalocyanine (CoPc) reduces the potential for electro-oxidation reactions of many chemical species (Roth et al. 2010), also having a high chemical and thermal stability. Thus, it can be used in electrocatalytic processes.

Many studies recently are using CN modified with CoPc for determination of several analytes, such as ascorbic acid (Zuo et al. 2012), hydrogen peroxide (Wang et al. 2015) epinephrine (Moraes et al., 2010), guanine (Balan et al. 2012), bisphenol A (YIN et al. 2010) and formic acid (Zeng et al. 2014). Another analyte that may be determined is L-Dopa.

The L-Dopa (or levodopa) is a medicine used to treat Parkinson's disease patients. Parkinson's disease is a neurological disease that causes tremors and difficulty to walk, do jogging and coordinate. Nerve cells use a chemical called dopamine to help control muscle movement. Parkinson's disease arises due to decreased dopamine production (Faria et al. 2003).

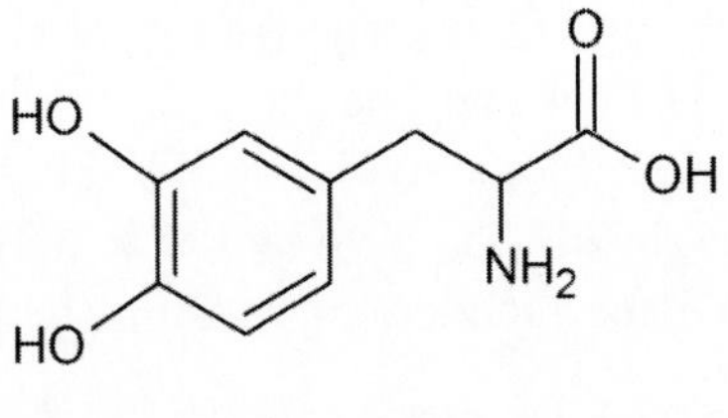

Figure 2. Structural formula of L-Dopa.

However, dopamine cannot be administered orally because it does not croos the blood-brain barrier. Thus, to stimulate dopamine production in the body, L-Dopa is administered since it is a precursor of dopamine. L-Dopa is converted into dopamine (Figure 2) by the *enzyme* dopa decarboxylase compensating her deficiency in the body (Bergamini et al. 2005).

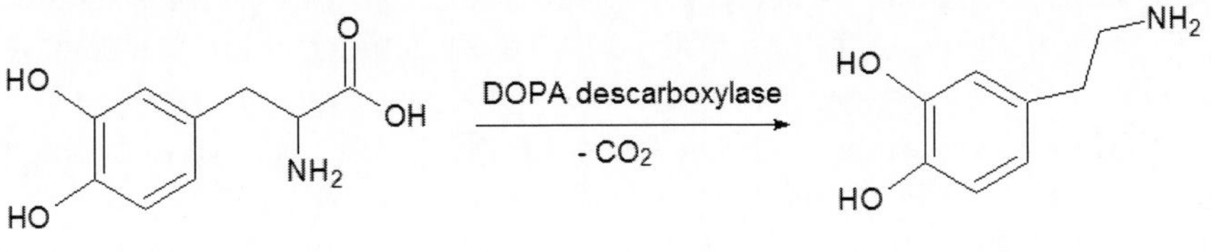

Figure 3. L-dopa conversion to dopamine by the enzyme dopa-decarboxylase.

Various methods can be used to determine the concentration of L-Dopa in pharmaceutical formulations, such as chromatography and spectrophotometry. However electrochemical techniques have been a good alternative since they have good precision and accuracy, high sensitivity and low cost. Among various electrochemical methods, voltammetry is an appropriate method for detecting organic compounds due to its simplicity and speed (Liu et al. 2003).

Recent studies have used CME to determine this drug. In 2011 Yan fabricated a cobalt hexacyanoferrate/large-mesopore carbon modified glassy carbon electrode (CoHCF–LMC/GC) by electrodepositing CoHCF film on LMC. The electrochemical behaviors of L-dopa at this modified electrode have been studied. Amperometry results depict that the proposed sensor provides excellent performance towards the determination of L-dopa with a low detection limit of 1.7 $\mu mol.L^{-1}$ (Yan et al. 2011).

In 2012 Leite et al. presented a sensitive and selective method for the voltammetric determination of L-Dopa in pharmaceutical formulations using a basal plane pyrolytic graphite (BPPG) electrode modified with chloro (pyridine)bis(dimethylglyoximato)cobalt(III) (Co(DMG)$_2$ClPy) absorbed in a multi-walled carbon nanotube (MWCNT). The results obtained were a detection limit of 0.86 $\mu mol.L^{-1}$ (Leite et al. 2012). Arvand et al. developed in 2014 an electrospun titanium dioxide nanofiber/graphite oxide paste/glassy carbon electrode for voltammetric determination of levodopa (l-DOPA) in aqueous media. As results presented good linear relationship with limit of detection of 15.94 $nmol.L^{-1}$ (Arvand et al. 2014).

This chapter aims to develop an electrochemical sensor in order to determine L-Dopa in pharmaceutical formulations using the voltammetry as technique. For this purpose , it was studied and optimized the concentration of the NC and the modifier CoPc. Besides optimize experimental conditions such as: pH, type of supporting electrolyte and its concentration, the effect of buffer system. The sensor was characterize for the following analytical parameters: selectivity, sensitivity, detection limit and linear response range. It was investigated which voltammetric technique have better sensitivity: cyclic voltammetry (CV), the differential pulse voltammetry (DPV) or square wave voltammetry (SWV). By the end the device developed was used for the determination of L-Dopa in real samples (pharmaceutical composition).

2. EXPERIMENTAL

2.1. Reagents and Solutions

All chemicals used were of analytical grade. The multi-wall carbon nanotubes (purity 99%, 6-13 nm diameter, 3.5-20 μm length) were acquired from Nanocyl. Cobalt(II) phthalocyanine, 3,4-Dihydroxy-L-phenylalanine (L-Dopa), Sodium hydroxide, Potassium chloride, 1,4-Piperazinediethane-sulfonic acid (PIPES), 4-(2-Hydroxyethyl)piperazine-1-ethanesulfonic acid (HEPES) and 2-Amino-2-(hydroxymethyl)-1,3-propanediol (Trizma) were purchased from Sigma-Aldrich®. Sodium chloride, dimethyl sulfoxide (DMSO), sodium phosphate monobasic, sodium phosphate dibasic, sodium sulfate and sodium nitrate were acquired from Synth. Lithium nitrate and hydrochloric acid was obtained from

Dinâmica® Química. Prolopa® (100/25 mg) was purchased from Roche. All solutions were prepared with deionized water purified Milli-Q® Integral Water Purification System. The actual ph of the buffer solutions was determined with a phmeter Tecnal TEC-50 and was adjusted with 0.1 mol.L-1 hydrochloric acid and 0.1 mol.L-1 sodium hydroxide.

2.2. Preparation of the Modified Electrode

A glassy carbon electrode (GCE) of geometric area of 0.071 cm^2 was used in the presented chapter. The alumina was used as an abrasive for cleaning of the electrode surface. The surface was thoroughly washed.

In order to modify the electrode surface, a 10 µL aliquot of the suspension containing CoPc and MWCN was added on the surface, leaving it to dry at 60° C for about 20 minutes. The concentrations of MWCN and CoPc were varied in order to optimize it. The suspension MWCN/CoPc was prepared by dispersing the materials in dimethylsulfoxide, using ultrasound.

2.3. Material Characterization and Electrochemical Measurements

Electrochemical measurements were performed with an Autolab PGSTAT12 potentiostat/galvanostat from Ecochemie coupled to a PC microcomputer with NOVA 1.8 software. A three-electrode electrochemical cell was employed for all electrochemical measurements. The electrodes were inserted into a 10 mL beaker through holes. The working electrode was a modified GCE. The auxiliary and reference electrodes were a platinum wire and Ag/AgCl, respectively.

Scanning Electron Micrographs (SEM) were obtained using a JEOL JSM-6510LV Scanning Electron Microscope. Fourier Transform Infrared (FT-IR) spectra was carried out on a UV–Vis-NIR Cary-5000 spectrometer.

2.4. Preparation and Electrochemical Analysis of Pharmaceutical Samples

The electrochemical behavior of the developed sensor was evaluated using cyclic voltammetry. It evaluated the factors that influence the charge transfer process between the electron mediator and the surface of the electrodes, such as the pH of the solution, the effect of supporting electrolyte, the buffer solution, scan rate and proportion of modifier (MWCN/CoPc).

To determine the best technique to be used for determining L-Dopa, the operating parameters of the differential pulse voltammetry (scan rate and pulse width) and square wave voltammetry (amplitude and pulse rate) were optimized. After an analytical curve was constructed for each techniques and sensitivity between them was compared.

For recovery studies, a concentration solution of 0.01 mol.L^{-1} of L-Dopa using a commercial sample was prepared. Then 50 µmol.L^{-1} of this solution was added to the electrochemical cell for the recovery studies.

3. RESULTS AND DISCUSSION

3.1. Electrochemical Behavior of L-Dopa

The electrochemical behavior of L-Dopa at glassy carbon electrode with and without the modification was investigated using cyclic voltammetry (CV) at buffer system pH = 7.0. The cyclic voltammograms obtained for L-Dopa 1.0 mmol.L^{-1} at glassy carbon electrode exhibit a well-defined anodic peak at a potencial of 420 mV.

The results are shown in Figure 4, where it can be seen that when using CGE/CoPc/MWCN in the presence of L-Dopa there is a significant reduction in oxidation potential of L-Dopa from 420 mV to about 180 mV. It is observed a significant increase in the analyte oxidation current. Thus, this result suggests that the modifier (carbon nanotubes with cobalt phthalocyanine) produces catalysis of L-dopa oxidation reaction.

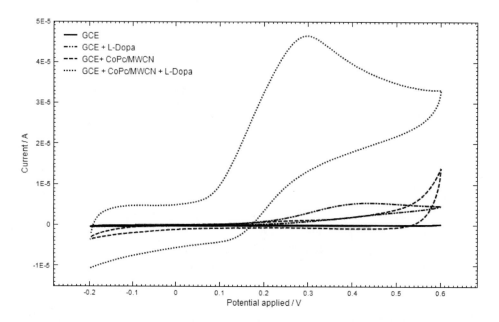

Figure 4. Cyclic *voltammograms*: glassy carbon electrode in the presence and absence of L-Dopa 1.0 mmol.L^{-1}; and glassy carbon electrode modified with MWCN/CoPc the presence and absence of L-Dopa 1.0 mmol.L^{-1}.

3.2. Morphology and Structure Characterizations

In order to analyze the morphology and composition of CoPc and MWCN, before and after modification with CoPc, the caractherization was performed by Scanning Electron Microscopy measures (SEM). The Figure 5a shows the image of MWCN before modification in order to compare with the others scans. As in Figure 5b it observed that in the absence of MWCN deposits with large aggregates of CoPc in the surface of the GCE are formed. It was observed in Figure 5c that CoPc molecules are distributed over the MWCN without forming large aggregates, showing a homogeneous distribution.

In order to identify the components in a mixture of the CoPc, MWCN and MWCN/CoPc, the samples were analyzed by Fourier transform infrared spectroscopy (FT-IR).

The absorption spectrum of MWCN at Figure 6a shows a band at 3419 cm^{-1} assigned to the stretching of carboxyl groups on the surface of carbon nanotubes (O = C - OH and C - OH) and the stretch of the hydroxyl groups. (Gupta et al. 2011).

Verma et al. in 2008 established the reference values of peaks in the FT-IR spectrum of CoPc. In the Figure 6b the spectrum for CoPc showed a large number of peaks between 768 cm^{-1} and 1613 cm^{-1}. Comparing them with the values established there is evidently the nature of CoPc. The peak at 1613 cm^{-1} is attributed to the ring deformation C=C and in 1525 cm^{-1} to stretching of C=N bond. The peaks in 1122 and 1088 cm^{-1} are attributed to deformation of C-H bond in-plane and in 738 cm^{-1} to deformation of C-H bond out-of-plane (Verma et al. 2008).

Then in the Figure 6c peaks and bands corresponding to both MWCN and CoPc are observed, showing that the material is composed of these two compounds. These result are desired because certify that the CoPc is adsorbed in the MWCN on the developed sensor.

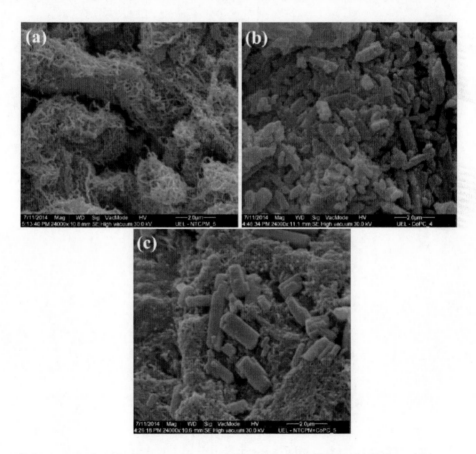

Figure 5. Images obtained by Scanning Electron Microscopy (a) MWCN, (b) CoPc and (c) MWCN/CoPc.

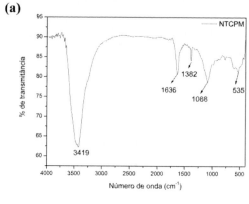

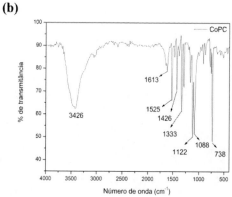

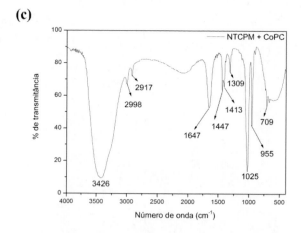

Figure 6. FT-IR spectrum for (a) MWCN, (b) CoPc and (c) MWCN/CoPc.

3.3. Influence of Scan Rate and Electrochemical Characterization

The influence of the scan rate in the developed system MWCN/CoPc is shown (Figure 7).

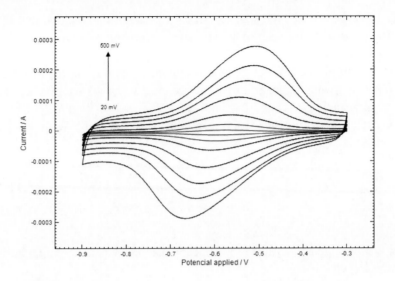

Figure 7. Cyclic voltammograms for GCE/CoPc/MWCN in phosphate buffer 0.01 mol.L^{-1} pH 7.5 in scan rate range of 20 - 500 mV.s^{-1}.

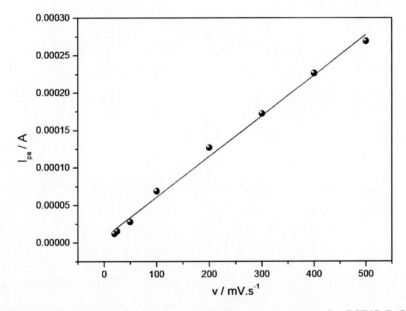

Figure 8. Dependence of the anodic peak current density *versus* scan rate for GCE/CoPc/MWCN in phosphate buffer 0.01 mol.L^{-1} pH 7.5 in scan rate range of 20 - 500 mV.s^{-1}.

It is possible to confirm a redox couple assigned to Co^{I}Pc/Co^{II}Pc with average potential at -585 mV. This influence is explained due to a reversible electron transfer reaction in terms of the diffusion and layer thickness.

Additionally, the study of the oxidation current peak *versus* the variation of the scan rate in the range of 20 - 500 mV.s^{-1} resulted in a linear relationship that is characteristic of the surface-redox process.

In order to study the electron transfer kinetics between the solution and the electrode surface, parameters such as α (electron transfer coefficient) and κ (heterogeneous transfer rate constant) were estimated.

The electron transfer coefficient (α) was estimated by evaluating the behavior of anodic and cathodic potential with the logarithm of the scan rate using the Laviron method (Laviron, 1979). For high scan rates values, E_{pa} and E_{pc} *versus* log v (Figure 9) becomes linear. Through the following expressions, the coefficients (α_a and α_c) were calculated using equations 1 and 2:

$$|s_a| = +\frac{2,3RT}{\alpha_a nF}$$ Equation (1)

$$|s_c| = -\frac{2,3RT}{\alpha_c nF}$$ Equation (2)

where s_a e s_b are the angular coefficients for linear equations obtained through the relationship E_{pa} e E_{pc} *versus* log v.

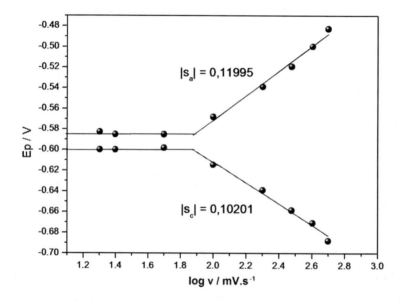

Figure 9. Effect of potential behavior of anodic and cathodic peak with the logarithm of the speed for GCE/CoPc/MWCN in phosphate buffer 0.01 mol.L^{-1} pH 7,5.

Since that two electrons (n) are involved in the redox reaction and that R is the gas constant (8.314 J.K^{-1}.mol^{-1}), T the absolute temperature (298.15 K) and F the Faraday constant (96485.34 C.mol^{-1}). The average value for coefficient α_a was 0.54.

The heterogeneous transfer rate constant (κ) was calculated using the equation 3:

$$\kappa = \frac{\alpha nFv}{RT}$$ Equation (3)

The heterogeneous transfer rate constant for scan rate (v) of 1,0 V.s^{-1} was 22,55 s^{-1}. These results suggest that the CoPc immobilized on GCE/MWCN form quasi-reversible with high transfer speed response. Indicating that the sensor is kinetically viable for electrooxidation of CoPc, enabling its use as a catalyst for redox processes of various electroactive species.

3.4. L-Dopa Electrochemical Oxidation on GCE/MWCN/CoPc

In this study of electrochemical oxidation of L-Dopa on the modified electrode, the variation of the anodic peak current *versus* scan rate was analysed. According to Andrieux and Saveant (Andrieux et al. 1978) the anodic peak current is proportional to the square root of the scan rate as shown in the following equation 4:

$$I_P = 0{,}496FAC_RD_R^{\frac{1}{2}}\left(\frac{Fv}{RT}\right)^{\frac{1}{2}}$$ Equation (4)

Since C_R = concentration of the analyte; D_R = diffusion coefficient of the analyte; F = Faraday constant; R = gas constant; T = temperature.

It can be observed a linear correlation by plotting a graphic of the anodic peak potential *versus* square root of scan rate (Figure 10).

This linearity on the graphic indicates that reaction is limited by mass transport, typical feature of electrocatalytic processes. Thus, these results show that the electrochemical oxidation of L-Dopa, in the GCE/MWCN/CoPc, can be controlled by diffusion of L-Dopa solution.

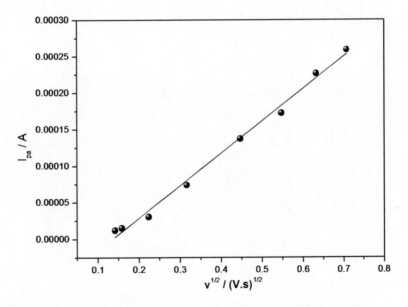

Figure 10. Dependence of the anodic peak current density and the square root of scan rate for GCE/CoPc/MWCN in phosphate buffer 0.01 mol.L^{-1} pH 7.5 in L-Dopa 1.0 mmol.L^{-1}.

3.5. Effect of Concentration of MWCN and CoPc in the Developed Sensor

It was studied the factors that influence the charge transfer process between the molecules of the modifier and the electrode surface. The first factor is the concentration of MWCN and CoPc that will be used to modify the electrode surface. For this matter, the sensitivity in each different concentration were compared . The results are shown below (Figure 11). In Figure 11a it can emphasize that a greater sensitivity appears on MWCN concentration equal to 2.0 mg.mL^{-1}. At lower concentrations, it is possible that it is not sufficient to completely immobilize the catalyst. As at higher concentrations, the excess may cause a blockage of the catalytic sites of cobalt phthalocyanine.

About the CoPc in Figure 11b the concentration of 2.0 to mg.mL^{-1} presented a higher sensitivity and it was used in subsequent studies. A higher concentration may not be sufficient to completely immobilize the catalytic site of cobalt phthalocyanine by the MWNC, that can cause a reduction of the sensor sensitivity.

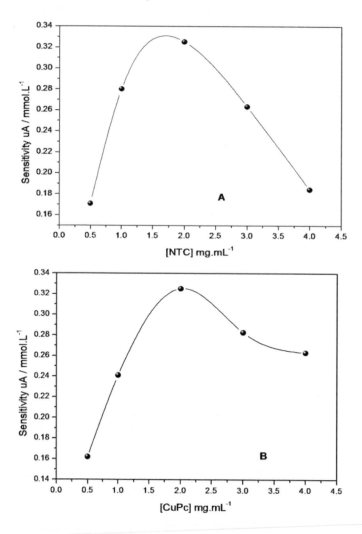

Figure 11. Influence of concentration of MWCN (a) and CoPc (b) in the modifier on the anodic peak current for L-DOPA oxidation of the chemically modified electrode.

3.6. Effect of Buffer Composition, Buffer Concentration and pH on the Oxidation of L-Dopa

To date, all studies were performed with phosphate buffer as supporting electrolyte. Thus, in order to evaluate the influence that the buffer type has on the electrochemical response, HEPES, TRIZMA and PIPES buffer solutions were prepared at a concentration of 0.1 mol.L^{-1} and pH 7.0, and the studies were conducted using the cyclic voltammetry.

Furthermore, in order to evaluate the effect of cations and anions, solutions were prepared with different cations and anions. It was found to peak separation and the formal potential for all electrolytes. The results can be seen in Figure 12.

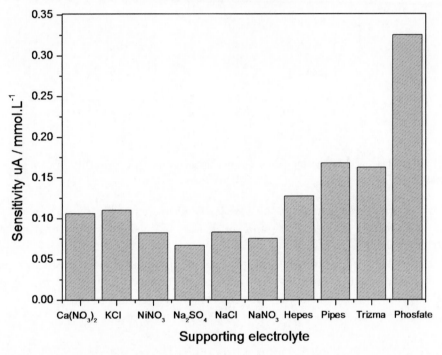

Figure 12. Supporting electrolyte influence on the anodic peak current for L-DOPA oxidation of the chemically modified electrode.

Sensitivity data for all electrolytes investigated presented similar results. Probably the electrolytes do not interact in such strong way with the electrode surface. Regarding buffer systems, the results were superior for sensitivity probably for providing greater system stability. Then according to these data show, the process that has the best response is phosphate buffer where the system has greater sensitivity. This behavior may be related to the interaction of phosphate buffer molecules with the modifier. The influence of pH on the modified electrode MWCN/CoPc behavior was also investigated using as support electrolyte phosphate buffer solution 0.1 mol.L^{-1} in a pH range between 5.5 and 8.5 (Figure 13).

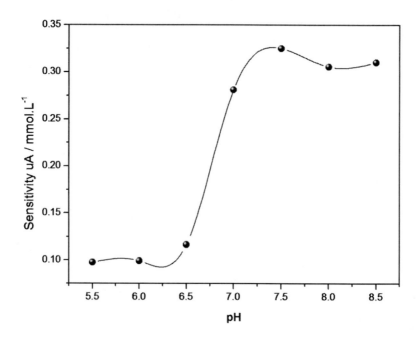

Figure 13. Influence of pH of the support electrolyte anodic peak current for L-DOPA oxidation on the chemically modified electrode.

The results show an increase in sensitivity when it increases pH in the range between 5.5 and 7.5. After the pH 7.5 were no significant changes in sensitivity. Therefore, the latter was used for other studies.

Finally, it analyzed the influence of the concentration of supporting electrolyte presented on the proposed system (Figure 14). Thus, the results obtained in the performed studies, the optimal experimental parameters of the GCE/MWCN/CoPc are in the following Table 1. Reminding that all studies ahead were performed using these parameters.

Table 1. Optimal experimental parameters

Experimental Parameters	Optimized Value
NC Concentration	2 mg.mL^{-1}
CoPc Concentration	2 mg.mL^{-1}
Supporting Electrolyte	Phosffate Buffer
pH of Supporting Electrolyte	7.5
Electrolyte Concentration	0.1 mol.L^{-1}

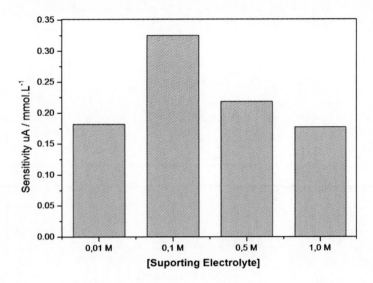

Figure 14. Influence of concentration of supporting electrolyte on the anodic peak current for L-DOPA oxidation on the chemically modified electrode.

3.7. Analytical Curve Obtained by Cyclic Voltammetry (CV)

After optimization of experimental parameters, an analytical curve for L-DOPA was obtained. Figure 15 shows the cyclic voltammograms obtained from successive additions of L-Dopa to the electrochemical cell. The analytical curve for L-DOPA obtained with the proposed sensor showed a linear response range between 110 and 270 μmol.L^{-1}, which can be expressed according to Equation 5, with sensitivity equal to 0.05025 μA/μmol.L^{-1}.

$$I\ (\mu A) = -0.69017 + 0.05025\ [\text{L-Dopa}/\mu\text{mol.L}^{-1}] \qquad \text{(Equation 5)}$$

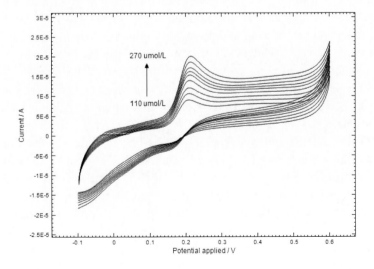

Figure 15. (Continued).

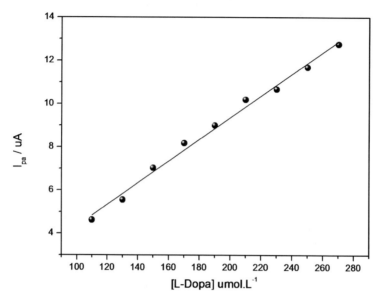

Figure 15. (a) Cyclic voltammograms in phosphate buffer containing L-Dopa in the concentrations: 110 - 270 umol.L^{-1}. (b) Analytical curve for the data of Figure 15a GCE/MWCN/CoPc in 0.1 mol.L^{-1} phosphate buffer pH 7.5 v = 20 mV.s^{-1} using cyclic voltammetry as technique.

3.8. Optimization of Operating Parameters of the Techniques of Square Wave Voltammetry (SWV) and Differential Pulse Voltammetry (DPV)

In SWV a symmetrical square wave is superimposed on a staircase waveform where the forward pulse of the square wave (pulse direction same as the scan direction) is coincident with the staircase step. The current is sampled twice during each square wave cycle, one at the end of the forward pulse, and again at the end of the reverse pulse (Christie et al. 1977).

The difference current between the two measurements is plotted *versus* the potential staircase. Square wave voltammetry yields peaks for faradaic processes, where the peak height is directly proportional to the concentration of the species in solution. (Favaron 1998). Thus, the frequency and the pulse amplitude are very important parameters in the SWV, since determine the signal strength, which is directly related to sensitivity of the technique. So the frequency was initially varied in the range of 10 to 100 Hz, while keeping fixed amplitude 25 mV. After the frequency with the highest sensitivity was fixed and amplitude was varied (10 mV - 100 mV). All voltammograms were obtained in solution containing 1 mmol.L^{-1} of L-Dopa in phosphate buffer solution 0.1 mol.L^{-1} (pH 7.5), with the use of the GCE/MWCN/CoPc under conditions experimental optimized. After que parameters of SWV were optimized, the parameters of DPV were studied. The current is measured before the application of the pulse (S1) and after application (S2), then the difference is registered between the two chains against the applied potential and the resulting voltammogram has the shape of a gaussian curve whose height is proportional to concentration of the analyte (Pessoa, 2001). On the DPV the scan rate and pulse amplitude are important parameters because they are directly related to sensitivity and selectivity. Thus, the initial scan rate was varied in the range from 2 to 50 mV.s^{-1}, keeping constant the amplitude 25 mV. After the optimized speed was kept constant and the amplitude was varied (10 mV - 100 mV).

Table 2. Summary of conditions optimized for SWV and DPV

Technique	Frequency	Pulse Amplitude	Scan Rate
SWV	10 Hz	10 mV	---
DPV	---	50 mV	50 mV/s

Thus, the operating parameters of the two electroanalytical techniques (DPV and SWV) were optimized (Table 2).

3.9. Analytical curves obtained by Square Wave Voltammetry (SWV) and Differencial Pulse Voltammetry (DPV)

Figure 16 shows the voltammograms obtained from successive additions of L-Dopa to the electrochemical cell using SWV as technique. The analytical curve-for L-DOPA obtained with the proposed sensor showed a linear response range between 10 and 150 µmol.L^{-1}, which can be expressed according to Equation 6, with sensitivity equal to 0.09728 µA/µmol.L^{-1}.

$$I (\mu A) = 1.52026 + 0.009728 \ [\text{L-Dopa/}\mu mol.L^{-1}] \qquad \text{(Equation 6)}$$

And the Figure 17 shows the voltammograms obtained using the DPV as a technique. The analytical curve for L-DOPA obtained exhibited a range of linear response between 10 and 80 µmol.L^{-1}, which can be expressed according to Equation 7, with sensitivity equal to 0.2877 uA/µmol.L^{-1}.

$$I (\mu A) = 0.09664 + 0.28768 \ [\text{L-Dopa/}\mu mol.L^{-1}] \qquad \text{(Equation 7)}$$

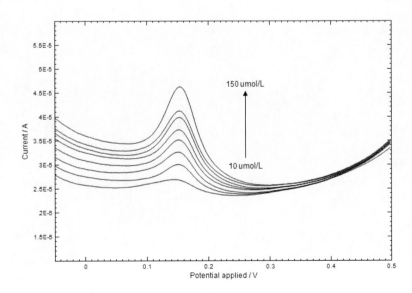

Figure 16. (Continued).

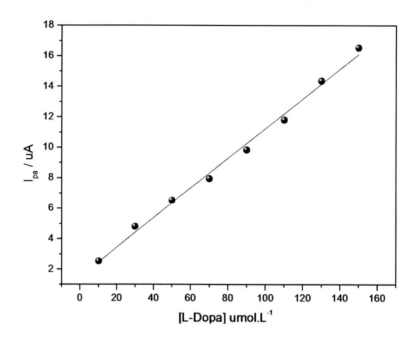

Figure 16. (a) Square wave voltammograms in phosphate buffer containing L-Dopa in the following concentrations: 10 - 130 umol.L^{-1}. (b) Analytical curve for the data of Figure 18a GCE/MWCN/CoPc in 0.1 molL^{-1} phosphate buffer pH 7.5 v = 20 mV.s^{-1} using square wave voltammetry as technique.

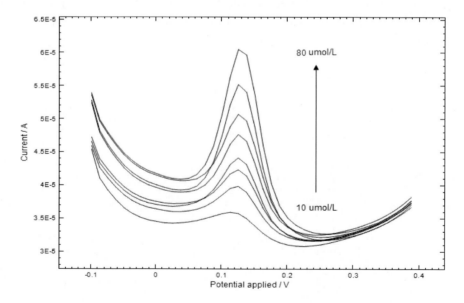

Figure 17. (Continued).

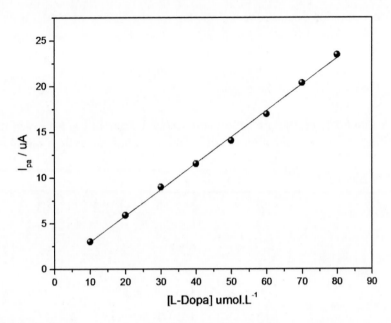

Figure 17. (a) Differential pulse voltammograms in phosphate buffer containing L-Dopa in the following concentrations: 10 - 80 umol.L^{-1}. (b) Analytical curve for the data of Figure 19a GCE/MWCN/CoPc in 0.1 molL^{-1} phosphate buffer pH 7.5 v = 20 mV.s^{-1} using differential pulse voltammetry as technique.

Since the differential pulse voltammetry showed a higher sensitivity, showing well defined peaks, it was chosen for use in the determination of L-Dopa in pharmaceutical formulations.

3.10. Validation of Analytical Method

The development of an analytical method, adapting or implementing a method involves the evaluation process to estimate their efficiency in laboratory routine. This process is usually called validation (Brito et al. 2003). Validation is a systematic process, through experimental studies, ensures that the method is in accordance with the requirements of the analytical applications, ensuring the reliability of results. (Ribani et al. 2004).

In Brazil, laboratories that perform chemical analysis should undergo an accreditation at approved agencies such as ANVISA (National Health Surveillance Agency) and INMETRO (National Institute of Metrology, Standardization and Industrial Quality) that provide validation of analytical methods guides (Brito et al. 2003). The analytical parameters called figures of merit, usually found for validation of analytical methods are: sensitivity, linearity, precision, accuracy, limit of detection (LOD), limit of quantification (LOQ).

Validation studies in this chapter were carried out taking into account the Resolution No. 899 of ANVISA. Linearity was assessed by analysis of the analyte in triplicate at concentrations of 42.5, 45.0, 47.5, 50.0, 52.5, 55.0, 57.5 μmol.L^{-1}. The construction of the analytical curve was made by plotting a graph of the concentration of L-Dopa (μmol.L^{-1}) in the X axis *versus* the change in current (μA) for each concentration in Y axis. coefficients, angular and linear axis are obtained from this regression curve. This curve showed a linear response in concentration range from 42.5 to 57.5 $\mu mol.L^{-1}$ (80% to 120% of the theoretical concentration used from L-Dopa in pharmaceutical samples), with correlation coefficients greater than 0,99 for n = 8. The results for limits of detection and quantification were obtained and the relative standard deviation (RSD) is less than 5%.

Table 3 shows the results of these studies summarized.

Table 3. Linearity, limit of detection and quantification of the proposed method obtained in the determination of L-Dopa in pharmaceutical samples

Figures of Merit	Day	Results
Linear Equation*	1	Ipa = -13.21282 + 4.17663[L-Dopa]
	2	Ipa = -11.41205 + 0.37783[L-Dopa]
Correlation Coefficient	1	0.9973
	2	0.9986
Concentration Range	1	42.5 - 57.5 $\mu mol.L^{-1}$
	2	42.5 - 57.5 $\mu mol.L^{-1}$
LD ($\mu mol.L^{-1}$)	1	2.7022
	2	2.8037
LQ ($\mu mol.L^{-1}$)	1	9.0075
	2	9.3459

*Analytical curve plotted were performed with triplicate values.

Table 4. Precision and accuracy of the proposed method obtained in the determination of L-Dopa in pharmaceutical samples

Figures of Merit	Day	Concentration ($\mu mol.L^{-1}$)		
Theoretical Concentration		45.0	50.0	55.0
Interday (n^d = 2)				
Recovered Concentration	1	45.24	49.03	54.21
	2	45.27	49.20	55.19
Precision (RSD%)	1	0.31	0.26	0.27
	2	0.27	0.24	0.24
Accuracy (RE%)	1	1.00	1.45	0.75
	2	1.01	1.44	0.67
Intraday (n^a = 2)				
Recovered Concentration		45.25	49.11	54.70
Precision (RSD%)		0.29	0.25	0.26
Accuracy (RE%)		1.00	1.45	1,45

* n^d = number of days; n^a = number of replicates.

The intraday precision was performed in triplicate by means of the analysis of L-Dopa standard solution for three different levels of concentration of analytical curve: low (45.0 μmol.L^{-1}), medium (50.0 μmol.L^{-1}) and high (55.0 μmol.L^{-1}). The interday precision and accuracy were obtained during routine operation of the system described, for two consecutive days. The precision of the method was assessed by relative standard deviation (RSD%), while the accuracy was expressed by the percentage of the relative error (RE%). Table 4 presents a summary of these results.

The precision and accuracy values obtained in method validation showed on Table 3 and 4 were less than 5% maximum recommended by Resolution No. 899 of ANVISA. Therefore, proposed method for determination of L-Dopa was considered accurate and able to be applied to real samples.

3.11. Application in Pharmaceutical Formulations

The proposed sensor GCE/MWNT/CoPc was tested in pharmaceutical formulation containing the active compound (L-Dopa). A L-Dopa solution was prepared using the drug sample (Prolopa®) in the concentration of 50 μmol.L^{-1}. The results are presented in Table 5.

Table 5. Determination of L-Dopa concentration in pharmaceutical formulation

Measure	[L-Dopa] theoretical	[L-Dopa] recovered	Recovery %	RSD %
1	50 μmol.L^{-1}	49.25 μmol.L^{-1}	98.50	
2	50 μmol.L^{-1}	49.32 μmol.L^{-1}	98.64	
3	50 μmol.L^{-1}	49.59 μmol.L^{-1}	99.18	
Average	**50 μmol.L^{-1}**	**49.05 μmol.L^{-1}**	**98.77**	**0.35907**

The values were compared to 100% of L-Dopa and the values obtained showed satisfactory precision and accuracy, as shown by the great recoveries and relative standard deviation (RSD).

Analyses were performed in triplicate and the mean of the results obtained was 98.97% specification on the label of the drug. Thus, it can be concluded that the proposed method is an excellent alternative for the determination of L-Dopa in pharmaceutical formulations can be applied to quality control of this drug. Furthermore, the absence of sample pretreatment is very useful because it reduces the time of analyses and make it easier the application of the sensor.

CONCLUSION

This chapter showed that the glassy carbon electrode modified with MWCN/CoPc is a viable alternative to the analytical determination of L-Dopa in pharmaceutical formulations. It can, thus, be used for quality control in the pharmaceutical industry.

The morphology and structure characterization showed that MWCN and CoPc form a composite material, without formation of large agglomerates. The results further from electrochemical caracterization suggested that the CoPc immobilized on the GCE form a quasi-reversible with high transfer speed response. Thus demonstrating that the sensor is designed to kinetically feasible electrooxidation CoPc, enabling its use as a catalyst for redox processes various electroactive species.

It was possible to check that the redox couple assigned to $Co^IPc/Co^{II}Pc$ is explained due a reversible electron transfer reaction in terms of the diffusion layer thickness. The oxidation of L-Dopa is limited by mass transport, typical feature of electrocatalytic processes. The electrochemical oxidation of L-Dopa, in the GCE/MWCN/CoPc, can be controlled by diffusion of L-Dopa solution.

Moreover, optimization of the electrochemical techniques and experimental parameters provided the construction of a sensor with greater sensitivity. Since the differential pulse voltammetry had a higher sensitivity, providing obtaining well defined peaks, it was chosen for use in the determination of L-Dopa in pharmaceutical formulations.

The precision and accuracy values obtained in method validation presented by the developed sensor were less than 5% maximum recommended by Resolution No. 899 of ANVISA. Therefore, proposed method for determination of L-Dopa was considered accurate and able to be applied to real samples.

Applied to real samples, the values were compared to 100% of L-Dopa and the values obtained showed satisfactory precision and accuracy, as shown by the great recoveries and relative standard deviation (RSD). Thus, it can be concluded that the proposed method is an excellent alternative for the determination of L-Dopa in pharmaceutical formulations and, then, can be applied to quality control of this drug.

ACKNOWLEDGMENTS

The authors would like to thank the the Brazilian agencies Fapemig and Rede Mineira de Química for the financial support. Also Prof. Dr. César Ricardo Teixeira Tarley for the colaboration in morphology and structure characterizations.

REFERENCES

Amarante J.; Caldas, E. P. A.; Brito, N. M.; Santos, T. C. R.; Vale, M. L. B. F. Validação de métodos analíticos: uma breve revisão. *Cad. Pesq.*, 2001, 12, 116-131.

Andrieux, C. P.; Saveant, J. M.; *Journal of Electroanalytical Chemistry.* 1978, 93, 163.

Aryand, M.; Ghodsi, N. Electrospun TiO_2 nanofiber/graphite oxide modified electrode for electrochemical detection of l-DOPA in human cerebrospinal fluid. *Sensors and Actuators B: Chemical*, 2014, 204, 393-401.

Balan, I.; David, J. G.; David, V.; Stoica, A.; Mihailciuc, C.; Stamatin, I.; Ciucu, A. A. Electrocatalytic voltammetric determination of guanine at a cobalt phthalocyanine modified carbon nanotubes paste electrode. *Journal of Electroanalytical Chemistry*, 2011, 654, 8-12.

Bergamini, M. F.; Santos, A. L.; Stradiotto, N. R.; Zanoni, V. B. *Journal of Pharmaceutical and Biomedical Analysis*. 2005, 39, 54-59.

Brito, N. M.; Ozelito, P. A. J.; Polese, L.; Ribeiro, A. L. Validação de métodos analíticos: estratégia e discussão. *Pesticidas: R.Ecotoxicol. e Meio Ambiente*, Curitiba, 2003, 13, 129-146.

Canevari, T. C. (2008) *Ftalocianina de cobalto preparada in situ sobre o óxido misto SiO2/SnO2 obtido pelo processo sol-gel. Aplicação na oxidação eletrocatalítica do ácido oxálico e do nitrito* (Dissertação de Mestrado em Química Inorgânica). Instituto de Química – Unicamp.

Causon, R. Validation of chromatographic methods in biomedical analysis: viewpoint and discussion. J. *Chromatogr.*, 1997, 689, 175-180.

Christie, J. H.; Turner, J. A.; Oysteryoung, R. A. Square Wave Voltammetry at the Dropping Mercury Electrode: Theory. *Anal. Chem.*, 1977, 49, 1899.

Dias, S. L. P. (2003) *Utilização do material híbrido orgânico-inorgânico celulose óxido de titânio para a imobilização de alguns catalisadores* (Dissertação de Doutorado). Instituto de Química – Unicamp.

Faria W. M.; Filho Z. D.; Psiquiatria Biológica, 2003, 11 (2) 45-50.

Favaron, R. (1998) *Determinação voltamétrica de zinco e ferro em amostras eletrolíticas de galvanoplastia empregando-se eletrodo de mercúrio de gota estática e a técnica de voltametria de onda quadrada.* (Dissertação de Mestrado em Química Analítica) Instituto de Química – Unicamp.

Gupta, V. K.; Saleh, T. A.; Functionalization of tungsten oxide into MWCNT and its application for sunlight-induced degradation of rhodamine B. *Journal of Colloid and Interface Science*; 2011, 362, 337-344.

Herbst, M. H.; Macêdo, M. I. F.; Rocco A. M.; Tecnologia dos nanotubos de carbono: tendências e perspectivas de uma área multidisciplinar. *Química Nova*; Sociedade Brasileira de Química: São Paulo, SP, 2004, 27, 6.

Laviron, E.; *Journal of Electroanalytical Chemistry*. 1979, 101, 19.

Leite, F. R. F.; Maroneze, C. M.; Oliveira, A. B.; Santos, W. T. P.; Damos, F. S.; Luz, R. C. S. Development of a sensor for L-Dopa based on Co(DMG)2ClPy/multi-walled carbon nanotubes composite immobilized on basal plane pyrolytic graphite electrode. *Bioelectrochemistry*, 2012, 86, 22-29.

Liu, X.; Zhang, Z.; Cheng; G.; Dong, S.; *Electroanalysis*. 2003, 15(2), 103-107.

Moraes, F. C.; Golinelli, D. L. C.; Mascaro, L H.; Machado, S. A. S. Determination of epinephrine in urine using multi-walled carbon nanotube modified with cobalt phthalocyanine in a paraffin composite electrode. *Sensors and Actuators B: Chemical*, 2010, 148 492–497.

Morita, K..; Hirayama, N.; Imura, H.; Yamaguchi, A.; Teramae, N.; *Journal of Electroanalytical Chemistry*. 2011, 656, 192-197.

Pereira, A. C.; (2003) *Comportamento eletroquímico de alguns compostos orgânicos eletroativos imobilizados em suportes inorgânicos visando o desenvolvimento de sensores para NADH* (Tese de Doutorado em Química) Instituto de Química – Unicamp.

Pessoa, A. P. (2001) *Óxido de nióbio enxertado sobre a superfície da sílica gel: Preparação e utilização na construção de eletrodos modificados* (Tese de Doutorado em Química). Instituto de Química – Unicamp.

Ribani, M.; Bottoli, C. B. G.; Collins, C. H.; Jardim, I. C. S. F.; Melo, L. F. C. *Química Nova,* Sociedade Brasileira de Química: São Paulo, SP, 2004, 27, 771-780.

Roth, F.; König, A.; Kraus, R.; Grobosch, M.; Kroll, T.; Knupfer, M. Probing the molecular orbitals of FePc near the chemical potential using electron energyloss spectroscopy. *European Physical Journal B*, 13, 2010, 339-344.

Souza, D.; Machado, S.A.S.; Avaca, L. A.; Voltametria de onda Quadrada. Primeira parte: aspectos teóricos. *Química Nova,* Sociedade Brasileira de Química: São Paulo, SP, 2003, 26, 81-89.

Souza, M. F. B.; Eletrodos quimicamente modificados aplicados à eletroanálise: uma breve abordagem. *Química Nova,* Sociedade Brasileira de Química: São Paulo, SP, 1997, 20.

Todd, W.J.; Bailly, F.; Pavez, J.; Faguy, P.W.; Baldwin, R.P.; Buchanan, R.M. Electrochemically induced metalation of polymeric phthalocyanines. *Journal of the American Chemical Society*, 1998, 120, 4887-4888.

Verma, D.; Dasha, R.; Katti, K.S.; Schulz, D.S.; Caruso, A. N. Role of coordinated metal ions on the orientation of phthalocyanine based coatings. *Spectrochimica Acta Part A*, 2008, 70, 1180-1186.

Wang, H.; Bu, Y.; Dai, W.; Li, K.; Wang, H.; Zuo, W. X. Well-dispersed cobalt phthalocyanine nanorods on graphene for the electrochemical detection of hydrogen peroxide and glucose sensing. *Sensors and Actuators B: Chemical*, 2015, 216, 298-306.

Yan, X.; Pan, D.; Wang, H.; Bo, X.; Guo, L. Electrochemical determination of L-dopa at cobalt hexacyanoferrate/large-mesopore carbon composite modified electrode. *Journal of Electroanalytical Chemistry*, 2011, 663, 36-42.

Yin, H.; Zhou, Y.; Xu, J.; Ai, S.; Cui, L.; Zhu, L. Amperometric biosensor based on tyrosinase immobilized onto multiwalled carbon nanotubes-cobalt phthalocyanine-silk fibroin film and its application to determine bisphenol A. *Analytica Chimica Acta*, 2010, 659, 144-150.

Zeng, J.; Sun, S.; Zhong, J.; Li, X.; Wang, R.; Wu, L.; Wang, L.; Fan, Y. Pd nanoparticles supported on copper phthalocyanine functionalized carbon nanotubes for enhanced formic acid electrooxidation. *International Journal of Hydrogen Energy*, 2014, 39, 15928–15936.

Zuo, X.; Zhang, H.; Li, N. An electrochemical biosensor for determination of ascorbic acid by cobalt (II) phthalocyanine–multi-walled carbon nanotubes modified glassy carbon electrode. *Sensors and Actuators B: Chemical*, 2012, 161, 1074–107.

In: Pharmaceutical Formulation
Editor: Bruce Moore

ISBN: 978-1-63484-082-8
© 2015 Nova Science Publishers, Inc.

Chapter 4

ANTIMETASTATIC ACTIVITIES AND MECHANISMS OF ACTION AMONG BISDIOXOPIPERAZINE COMPOUNDS

Da-Yong Lu[1,2], Jian Ding[1], Rui-Ting Chen[1], Bin Xu[1] and Ting-Ren Lu[2]*

[1]Shanghai Institute of Materia Medica, Chinese Academy of Sciences, Shanghai, PR China
[2]Shanghai University, Shanghai, PR China

ABSTRACT

Bisdioxopiperazine compounds, including ICRF-154 and razoxane (ICRF-159, Raz), are anticancer agents developed in the UK in 1969. Novel discoveries and debates about these compounds have been frequently reported worldwide, especially the antimetastatic activity and detoxicatative for anticancer anthrocylines. Furthermore three bisdioxopiperazine derivatives (Biz compounds), bimolane (Bim), probimane (Pro) and MST-16, have been synthesized at the Shanghai Institute of Materia Medica, Chinese Academy of Sciences, PR China after 1980. Since cancer metastasis, the deadliest pathologic feature of cancers has been the main obstacle in cancer therapy, antimetastatic therapeutic efficacies and mechanisms of action about Biz compounds are of significant clinical interests of all time. This review addresses and highlights the different inhibitions against metastases *in vivo* and molecular mechanisms of action *in vitro* of Biz compounds especially relating to the inhibitory efficacies against tumor metastasis and other important clinical utilizations including inhibitory pathways against angiogenesis, topoisomerase II, calmodulin, sialic acid, fibrinogen, drug combinations, medicinal chemistry, cell-movement and so on. Since 90% cancer deaths are caused by neoplasm metastasis and cancer stem cells, the systematic exploration of antimetastatic activity and mechanisms of action for Biz compounds seems to be a shortcut for a final solution of cancer therapy in the future.

Keywords: Bisdioxopiperazine compounds, probimane, razoxane, MST-16, antimetastatic drugs, medicinal chemistry, angiogenesis, spontaneous metastases, drug combinations,

---

*Corresponding author: Dr Da Yong Lu, email: ludayong@sh163.net ludayong@shu.edu.cn.

calmodulin, sialic acids, fibrinogen, cell-movement, drug development, personalized cancer therapy

BACKGROUND

Cancer is one of the deadliest diseases that cause the 7-10 millions deaths annually worldwide (Ali et al., 2011(a), Ali et al., 2011(b), Siegel et al., 2015). Unlike cardiovascular diseases, the beneficiary outcome by clinical interventions for cancers especially for advanced cancer patients is improving slightly over the past several decades (Varmus 2006). Neoplasm metastasis is one of the deadly characters that are responsible for these unsatisfactory outcomes of cancer therapies and more than 90% of cancer deaths are caused by neoplasm metastasis and hopefully only controlled by effective drugs. Paradoxically to our efforts (billions of USD annually worldwide) and expectations (consistent financial or human resource supports in developed countries for more than half-century), unsatisfactory therapeutic benefits by present licensed antimetastatic drugs (usually antivascular or MMPs inhibitors) (Lu et al., 2013a) have been achieved until now. Therapeutic benefits in late-staged or aged cancer patients are especially poor and useless (Lu et al., 2013) and with some risks of toxicities by the applications of currently licensed antimetastatic drugs (Verheul and Pinedo 2007). Clinical anticancer drug therapies currently in use are mainly focusing on primary tumor growth rather than specifically targeting pathologic courses of metastases. An urgent requirement of finding important drugs targeting specifically to neoplasm metastases, metastatic cascade or formed metastatic nodule, is essential and indispensable. It nevertheless needs changing focus from targeting of vasculature and MMPs into other types antimetastatic drugs that target to other metastatic-relating molecules, pathways and personalized cancer therapy in clinics.

MEDICINAL CHEMISTRY AND THERAPEUTIC TARGETING INTRODUCTIONS OF BIZ COMPOUNDS

Biz compounds, including ICRF-154, razoxane (ICRF-159, *Raz*), ICRF-186 and ICRF-187 (two stereo-isomers of Raz) and ICRF-193, developed in the UK, were among the earliest agents found to be effective against a model of spontaneous metastasis (Lewis lung carcinoma) (Herman et al., 1982, Lu & Lu 2010a). (**Figure** 1) Ever since that time (1969) (Hellmann et al., 1969), many studies have addressed their potential use and mechanisms of action in clinical chemotherapy. Three main mechanisms of action have been investigated by widely repeated authors and therapeutic utilizations: potentiating the effect of radiotherapy, overcoming multi-drug resistance (MDR) to daunorubicin and doxorubicin in leukemia, and inhibiting topoisomerase II and so forth (Lu et al., 2004(b)). More importantly, *Raz* has been licensed in many countries as a cardioprotectant during anthrocycline treatment. (**Table** 1) (Lu et al., 2004b) Since Biz compounds are unique agents in their pharmacological mechanisms of action of metastases inhibition and are conservative anticancer and antimetastatic activities between Biz compounds, further medicinal chemistry or pharmacological studies seems indispensable and is of great medical significance. Thereafter, probimane (1,2-bis (N^4-morpholine-3, 5-dioxopiperazine-1-yl) propane; AT-2153, Pro) and MST-16 (1,2-bis (4-isobutoxycarbonyloxymethyl-3, 5-dioxopiperazin-1-yl) ethane) were synthesized at Shanghai Institute of Materia Medica, Chinese Academy of Sciences by Prof Yun-Feng Ren and Prof Jun-Cao Cai (Ji 1988, Lu & Lu 2010a).

The structural formulae of the three Biz compounds are represented in **Figure 1**. MST-16, as a licensed anticancer drug in Japan since 1994, is allowed for directly use in leukemia chemotherapy, mainly against adult T-cell leukemia (Okamoto et al., 2000).

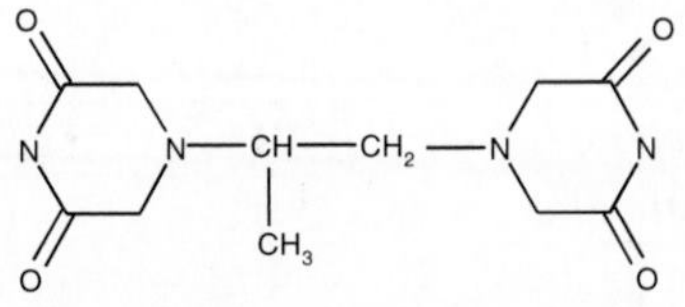

Razoxane

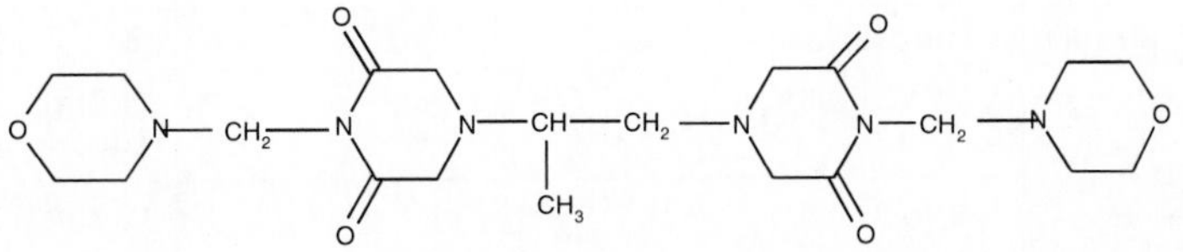

Probimane

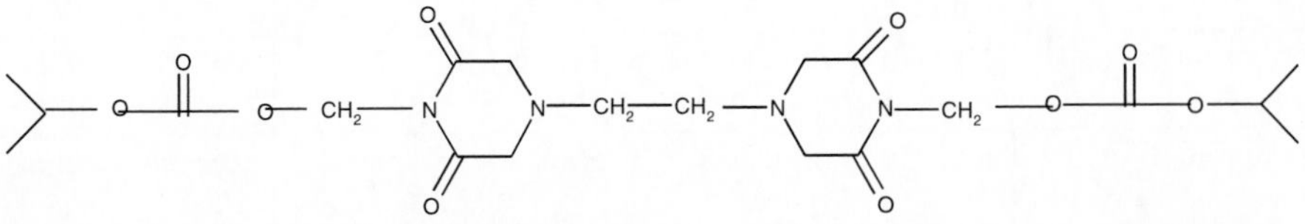

MST-16

Figure 1. Structural formulae of major bisdioxopiperazine compounds.

Experimental and Clinical Effectiveness of Biz Compounds

Experimental, clinical therapeutic efficacies and possible mechanisms of action of Biz compounds are outlined in **Table 1 and Table 2**. (Table 1 and Table 2) Many of these discoveries have been the clinical therapeutic options for Biz compound treatments. Among these therapeutic targets and applications, relieving the toxicities and MDR of anthrocyclines and metastatic inhibitions are the most famous ones. Besides, many other mechanisms and therapeutic targets for Biz compounds are documented. Among these mechanisms and therapeutic targets, neoplasm metastasis inhibitions are the most important ones.

Table 1. Major milestones and therapeutic efficacies of Biz compounds against tumor growths and metastases

Tumor types	Tumor model origin	Biz compounds	Reference sources
Sarcoma and leukemia	Murine tumor (in vivo)	ICRF-154 and Raz	Creighton et al., 1969
Pulmonary metastasis (LLC)	Murine tumors (in vivo)	Raz	Hellmann& Burrage 1969
Different human tumors	Clinical data	Raz	Bakowski, 1976
Colorectal tumors	Clinical data	Raz	Bellet et al., 1976
Malignant lymphoma	Clinical data	Raz	O'connel, 1980
Variety of tumors	Both animal and human tumors	Biz compounds	Herman et al., 1982
Leukemia	Murine tumor	MST-16	He et al., 1988
Ehrlich ascite	Murine tumor (in vitro)	Bim & Pro	Wang et al., 1988
Malignant lymphoma	Clinical data	Pro	Yang et al. 1990
Radiotherapy enhancement	Clinical data	Raz	Hellmann & Rhomberg 1991
Non-Hodgkin's lymphoma	Clinical data	MST-16	Okamoto et al., 2000
Pulmonary metastasis	Murine tumor (in vivo)	Pro	Lu et al., 2004b Lu et al., 2006
Lung tumor	Human tumor xenograft (in vivo)	Raz, Bim & Pro	Lu et al., 2004b
Variety of tumor cell lines	Human tumor (in vitro)	Pro & MST-16	Lu et al., 2005 Lu et al., 2006
Drug combination	Human tumor	Raz	Rhomberg et al., 2007
Different stage of metastatic cascade	Murine tumor (in vivo)	Raz, Bim and Pro	Lu & Lu, 2010a

Abbreviations. Raz—razoxane; Bim—bimolane, Pro—probimane.

Table 2. Mechanisms of action for Biz compounds against primary tumor growths

Drug-targeting molecules or pathways	Biz compounds	Reference sources
Tumor angiogenesis inhibitions	Most Biz compounds	Numerous references
Synergistic action with anthrocyclines	Most Biz compounds	Numerous references
Topoisomerase II inhibitions	ICRF-187 & ICRF-193	van Hille et al., 2000
Chromosome segregation block/ G_2M arrest	ICRF-187 & ICRF-193 Raz, Pro & MST-16 ICRF-154 & Bim	van Hille et al., 2000 Lu et al., 2005 Vuong et al., 2013
Calmodulin inhibition	Pro Raz & Pro	Lu et al., 2001 Lu et al., 2007c

Drug-targeting molecules or pathways	Biz compounds	Reference sources
Peroxidant inhibitions		Lu et al., 2003
GTPase/cell actin aggregation/ cell movements	Raz, Pro & MST-16	Lu & Lu, 2010b Lu et al., 2010c

Abbreviations. Raz—razoxane; Bim—bimolane; Pro—probimane.

Inhibitions on Neoplasm Metastases by Biz Compounds

90% cancer deaths are caused by neoplasm metastases owing to unknown mechanisms of action and targets of effective drugs (Lu et al., 2013a, Valastyan & Weinberg 2011). Biz compounds are the earliest anticancer agents found to especially inhibit spontaneous neoplasm metastases of Lewis lung carcinoma (LLC) (Hellmann et al., 1969, Lu et al., 2004b). Experimental metastasis models have been divided into two sub-categories— spontaneous metastatic models and artificial metastatic models. Artificial metastatic models usually inject tumor cells into the arteries or veins of hosting animals and finally metastasize in remote organs—mostly into lung of mice. Spontaneous metastatic models nevertheless encompass metastasize cascades of all natural ways in real human situations. From this theoretic opinion, Raz was regarded as a promising agent when it was first discovered. Since the inhibitory effect of Raz on spontaneous metastases is so strong, almost 90% of pulmonary metastatic foci are unrecognizable with a naked-eye after Biz compound treatment in mice bearing LLC (Hellmann et al., 1969, Lu et al., 2004b). A widely belief is thence that all metastases could be successively treated by Raz in all oncology circumstances. Surprisingly enough, clinical applications of Raz in the treatment of neoplasm metastases were widely discouraging. No significant survival benefit was found even after Raz treatment with formed neoplasm metastases (Herman et al., 1982). It is a great controversy that has been explained until recently (Lu et al., 2010a). As a consequence of this result, Raz has been controversy for being a commonly used antimetastatic agent worldwide.

The major pathways of antimetastatic activity of Biz compounds have been tabulated. (Table 3) Some detail information and references are discussed in the following sectors.

Spontaneous tumor metastases involve a fixed course of pathophysiological processes and are long pathogenesis processes to deteriorate the hosts in natural conditions, at least a week-long course in mice and a month-long course in human. It encompasses at least seven distinctive substages (1) invade locally through surrounding extracellular matrix (ECM) and stromal cell layers, (2) intravasate into the lumina of blood vessels; (3) tumor cells survive the rigors of transport through the vasculature; (4) arrest at distant organ sites; (5) tumor cells extravasate into the parenchyma of distant tissues; (6) initially survive in these foreign microenvironments in order to form micrometastases, and (7) reinitiate their proliferative programs at distant sites, thereby generating macroscopic, clinically detectable neoplastic growths (Lu et al., 2013a,Valastyan & Weinberg 2011). From anatomical and physiologic points of view, may the long-evolving course of a metastasis involve transitions through multiple organs and other tissues trigger diversified biochemical or molecular pathways in each substages (Lu et al., 2010a)? In this pathologic point of view, since the long-evolving course of a metastasis must travel more than one body-organ, the obvious anatomic differences of organs that carry malignant cells within a variety of metastasis stages, different molecules and pathways linking neoplasm metastases are possible (Lu et al., 2010a, Lu et al., 2013a).

Table 3. Major antimetastatic mechanisms of action and pathways involved by Biz compounds

Mechanisms and pathways	Biz compounds	Reference sources
Angiogenesis	Most of Biz compounds	Numerous articles
Tumor vasculature inhibitions	Raz	Salsbury et al. 1974
Tumor cells detached from primary tumor vessels	Raz	James & Salsbury, 1974
Enhanced drug accumulation in tumors/metastatic nodules	Pro	Lu et al., 1993 Lu et al., 2010b
Serum sialic acid inhibition in mice bearing tumors	Raz & Pro Pro	Lu et al., 1994 Lu et al., 2013b
Inhibiting the secretion of vascular factors in cancer patients	MST-16	Braybrooke et al., 2000
Calmodulin inhibition	Pro Pro	Lu et al., 2001 Lu et al., 2007c
Antioxidant efficacy	Raz & Pro	Lu et al., 2003
Inhibitions the binding of fibrinogen and tumor cells	Raz & Pro	Lu et al., 2004a
Different therapeutic efficacy among metastatic cascade	Raz, Bim & Pro	Lu et al., 2010 a
GTPase inhibition	Raz, Pro & MST-16	Lu & Lu, 2010 b
Tumor cell movement inhibitions *in vitro*	Raz, Pro & MST-16	Lu et al., 2010c

Abbreviations. Raz—razoxane; Bim—bimolane, Pro—probimane.

In return, different stage of metastatic cascades will certainly not be inhibited by a fixed type of drugs (Lu et al., 2010a, Lu et al., 2013a). Owing to these characteristics, the spontaneous metastatic inhibitory efficacies against LLC by a variety of Biz compounds are found to be different, especially between Raz and Pro (Lu et al., 2010a). Since the detachment of 3LL began at day 6-8 (James et al., 1974), therapeutic efficacies for formed pulmonary metastatic foci by Raz treatments later than day 8 might be obscured in this murine metastatic model (Lu et al., 2010a). However, Pro and Bim might be equally effective mice in formed metastatic foci of LLC. From our early data of ^{14}C-probimane tracing and autoradiography (Lu et al., 1993, Lu et al., 2010b), an obvious greater accumulation of Pro was found in tumor tissues, especially in metastatic foci. Since Raz can only inhibit the detachment of tumor cells from primary sites, yet less effective to tumor growths or metastasis themselves, cancer patients clinically undergoing chemotherapy (more than 50%) are conspicuous with metastasized tumors that Raz is less effective. Pro, nevertheless, might be useful in metastasis therapy according to this paradigm.

Biz compounds, especially Raz, has been originally regarded as agents to minimize blood vessels of tumors, however these blood vessels are thought to be an important step to support tumor growth and metastases (Braybrook 2000, Hellmann 2003, Salsbury et al., 1974). Apart from inhibitions on blood vessels in tumors, Raz has also been reported to inhibit vascular growth factors (Braybrook 2000). Since these kinds of reports are a multitude, there is no doubt that Biz compounds possess antivascular activities and related pharmaceutical functionalities. The slowdown of building blood capillary structures in tumors can explain the inhibition of the enlargements of metastatic nodule from small number cell congregations into noticeable metastatic foci. *Raz* and *Pro* show typical characteristics of antiangiogenesis agents, which target small nodule of tumors. However, this mechanism of actions of Raz is very similar to antivascular agents licensed worldwide, a common pathway antimetastatic drugs sharing and it lacks the originality in explaining the uniqueness of Biz compounds. It seems too hasty to be regarded as a sole and major pathway Biz compounds ought to act. Let us take it as one of the possibility to consider in the future.

NOVEL MECHANISMS OF ACTION

Due to small categories of advanced cancer patients are very effective by Biz compound treatments, a great deal of efforts, especially novel therapeutic mechanisms and medicinal chemistry investigations are urgently needed. Table 3 gives the overall information about this issue (Table 3).

Tumor Fibrinogen Pathways

Explanations of anticancer and antimetastatic mechanisms of *Biz* compounds are now inconclusive and commonplace (modern cliché) from other researchers. The present explanation for the anticancer mechanisms of action by *Raz* treatments is attributed to antiangiogenesis and topoisomerase II inhibition that are the universal pathways of many current anticancer drugs. Since the antimetastatic therapeutic activities of *Raz* and *Pro* were much stronger than those actions against primary tumor growth, the investigation on special targets of neoplasm metastasis ought to be more useful for laboratory and clinical cancer research and treatment study. In order to improve the therapeutic outcome, at first we must understand the key processes and molecular-relevance of metastatic cascade and testify more metastatic-related pathways and molecules. This work is of great clinical significant.

Fibrinogen is a century-long hot topic linked with tumor metastases (Bobek 2012, Costantini & Zacharski 1992, Dvorak et al., 1983, Grint et al., 2012, Lu et al., 2004a, Lu et al., 2007a, Lu, 2014, Lu et al., 2015). Experimental data suggest that there are three possible ways in which fibrinogen or fibrin may be involved in tumor growth and metastasis: (i) it may form a scaffold to which tumor cells can attach—as tumor stroma; (ii) it may form a tumor cocoon to shield tumor cells from attack by activated lymphocytes; (iii) it may help angiogenesis in tumor tissues (Costantini & Zacharski 1992, Dvorak et al., 1983).

Anticoagulants and fibrinolytic agents being used as assistant therapy for metastases have evolved for more than 4 decades (Bobek 2012, Lu et al., 2007a, Lu 2014, Lu et al., 2015). Fibrinogen and/ or fibrin, frequently occurring at the surrounding areas (matrix) of solid tumors, are regarded as a promoter for tumor growth and metastases. Patients with solid tumors often have high plasma fibrinogen level (Jones et al., 2006, Lu et al., 2000, Lu et al., 2007b, Polterauer et al., 2009). Therefore, many researchers have been working together for finding ways and strategies targeting fibrinogen around tumors—like using anticoagulants and fibrinolytic agents (Lu et al., 2007a, Lu 2014, Lu et al., 2015). In this work, it has been found that Pro and Raz, different from oxalysine, are no better than most of anticancer drugs in inhibiting fibrinogen coagulation (Lu et al., 1999), but, it has been recently found that Pro and Raz, along with most of the other anticancer drugs, may directly inhibit fibrinogen-tumor binding (Grint et al., 2012, Lu et al., 2004a). It changes our previous misconceptions that neoplasm metastases of fibrinogen-pathways can only be treated and controlled by anticoagulants, such as warfarin and heparin (Lu et al., 2007a). It created a new horizon of understanding and treatment of cancer metastases. Since we have found that Pro and Raz can inhibit the binding of fibrinogen to tumor cells (Lu et al., 2004a) *in vitro,* but enable to inhibit thrombin catalyzing of fibrinogen *in vitro,* it suggests that Pro and Raz are potentially selective agents in inhibiting fibrinogen-related or -targeted pathways and molecules and finally to be useful in cancer growth/metastasis treatments in both single agent and drug combinations.

Inhibition of Serum Sialic Acids in Mice Bearing Solid Tumors

Tumor metastasis is a foremost threat against theadvanced cancer patients in clinics. Many unfavorable molecules within or above tumor cells critically decide the pace and ranges of tumor spreading and metastases. One important type of biomolecules relating with neoplasm metastases is sialic acids (Lu & Cao 2001, Lu et al., 2011, Lu et al., 2012). Sialic acids are among the very few molecular categories that are found to be significant different between low- and high-metastatic tumor types and some of sialic acids are supposed to be only present in tumors (Lu & Cao 2001).

Our work shows that some of anticancer drugs, including Pro and Raz, can significantly inhibit serum sialic acid levels in mice bearing tumors S180 and Lewis lung carcinoma (Lu et al., 1994, Lu et al., 2013b). Of these anticancer drugs tested (more than ten), Pro is one of the most active anticancer drugs in inhibiting serum sialic acids (Lu et al., 2013b). Nevertheless, all these anticancer drugs can do nothing about the normal synthesis of sialic acids in non-tumor-bearing mice (Lu et al., 2013b).

Human Cell Calmodulin (CaM) Inhibitions

Calmodulin is a key molecule that decides and controls the growth and apoptosis of both normal and tumor cells. As a possible modulate, Pro has been found to inhibit the CaM activity on rabbit erythrocyte membranes (Lu et al., 2001, Lu et al., 2007c). We have also found the anti-CaM activity of Pro can be enhanced in the presence of sialic acids analogues (Lu et al., 2007c). As a counterpart of Pro, Raz has much less anti-CaM activity (Lu & Cao 2001). The reasons behind the scene must be further studied.

Since these findings are evident-oriented and have not been fully explained in molecular mechanisms of action bases, this is a seldom-studied target of therapeutic importance and can be a subject of more serious investigations in the future. However, our finding of inhibition of sialic acids in tumors by Biz compounds, especially by Pro is a good starting-point to this series of experimental and clinical studies. Further work can improve to build the relationship between CaM inhibitory efficacies and targeted therapeutic efficacy in the presence and absence of sialic acid step-by-step.

Anti-mobile Activity of Biz Compounds

Tumor cells invade and metastasize to surrounding or remote tissues through cell movements. Previous work also tackled this problem by two *in vitro* assays.

Anti-migration effects of Biz compounds against human mammary tumor cell lines, MDA-MB-435, for 24 h were evaluated by Matrigel migration assay (Lu et al., 2010c). Previously, it was found that Pro (1, 5 and 25µM) and MST-16 (5 and 50µM) inhibited tumor cell migration through Matrigel membrane. Pro at 25µM almost fully prevented MDA-MB-435 cells from entering into Matrigel membrane. Our finding suggested that Pro and MST-16 might reduce the numbers of tumors in Matrigel artificial membrane through inhibiting migration. Pro, MST-16 and ICRF-187 (2-5µM) inhibited human mammary tumor cell's (MDA-MB-435 and MDA-MB-468) movement significantly in wound-healing assay, almost active at the same dose range for inhibition of cell migration. (Lu et al., 2010c) With Biz-treatment for 24 h, though almost no tumor cells were found scattering in the cutting blank areas yet the control plate (no drugs present) was filled with tumor cells. These findings indicate that Biz compounds enable to block tumor cell from moving into the blank areas of plates (wound-healing). The effective dose range (1-5µM) of Biz compounds in this model is also much lower than their corresponding range in antiproliferate (IC_{50} >20µM) (Lu et al., 2005, Lu et al., 2010c). In addition, we have found that Pro, Raz and MST-16 at low concentrations can inhibit the GTPase activity of human mammary tumor cells (Lu & Lu 2010b), but show no change on ATPase activity of human mammary tumor cells. It is a good therapeutic potential for anti-move ability by Biz compound treatments. The proposed mechanisms of action (Biz compounds) are the cascade of GTPases inhibition to actin assembly slowdown to tumor cell movement control (Lu & Lu 2010b). This character is also explained for normal cell mutations for Biz compounds (ICRF-154 and bimolane) (Vuong et al., 2013).

In Vivo Distribution and Metabolisms of ^{14}C-Pro in Mice Bearing Tumors

The ^{14}C-labelled Pro was used to understanding the overall distribution and excretion of Pro in living bodies (Lu et al., 1993, Lu et al., 2010c), and the ^{14}C-labelled Pro distributed and excretions in different organs or tissues can be seen from our early reports (Lu et al., 1993, Lu et al., 2010b). A selective affinity and long-term accumulation of ^{14}C-Pro in tumor tissues (Lu et al., 1993, Lu et al., 2010b), especially in metastatic foci in lungs were firstly observed and reported by us (Lu et al., 2010b). It is therefore helpful to explain why the anticancer actions of Pro, especially selective inhibition against pulmonary metastases. It is shown that ^{14}C-labelled Pro is mainly excreted from both urine and feces in the similar profiles of rate and ratio in mice.

DISCUSSION

This work mainly has been focusing on the novel targets and pathways among Biz compounds for their antimetastatic action from laboratory data to translational work. In the past, the explanations for antimetastatic actions of Biz compounds focused on anti-angiogeneses and intermediation of tumor DNA rearrangement by topoisomerase II (Table 1-3). Generally speaking, most angiogenesis inhibitors are often low efficacies in cytotoxicity and hardly eradication of larger volumes of tumors such as low response to patients with large tumor volumes (solid tumors). Their therapeutic action is to control dormant metastatic cell congregation in diameter sizes less than 0.5 mm (Lu et al., 2013a). These kinds of agents will be better to combine with cytotoxic drugs clinically (Lu 2014). The higher antiproliferative effects and affinity to metastatic foci of probimane may decide its greater potentiality in future uses. More mechanisms of action need to be clarified in further study. Novel ideas have been initiated in following studies.

Since Biz compounds are not first-line anticancer drugs, they are mostly used as cardio-protective agents or venous leakages for anticancer anthrocycline (Kane et al., 2008) and sometimes as combinative agents for advanced cancer patients (Rhomberg et al., 2007). Owing to the small-range of clinical Biz compound application, no large-scale financial aid is supported. It leads to slow pace of experimental or clinical Biz compound studies. In order to learn more about the favorable or undesired characteristics of Biz compounds, more attentions should be paid for creating novel ideas and therapeutic mechanisms of action under tight budgets.

The most important aspects of Biz compound researches are to analyze and understand the novel molecular mechanisms of action against neoplasm metastases. The novel molecular targeting we proposed herein included pathways of inhibitions against sialic acids and fibrinogen. Though these kinds of shotgun-like approaches need to be reinforced, they do open a new realm and panorama of metastasis treatments. Within the realm of metastatic therapy, some new ideas and useful laboratory data (sialic acids, fibrinogen and cell movement) mainly studied in this lab are especially explained. We hope this work will be a good beginning for systematic study of antimetastatic activity of Biz compounds and create well-informed strategy for individualized cancer chemotherapy (Lu 2014).

This work indicates that Biz compounds inhibit tumor cell migration *in vitro* through Matrigel-Coated Transwells and evidence by a wound-healing assay in three human mammary tumor cell lines (Lu et al., 2010c). In searching for molecular targets for driving the movement inhibition by Biz compounds, it has been found that Pro, ICRF-187 and MST-16 affect the network of actin assembly and GTPase activity. This is new discovered pathways that may impact Biz compounds greatly and has therapeutic significance. By observations of all these new pathways, we have obtained clarified scenery and possibilities in Biz compounds metastatic therapies in clinics. We argue the systematic exploration of antimetastatic activity and mechanisms of Biz compounds seems to be a shortcut for a final solution of cancer therapy in the future.

NEW PERSPECTIVE

Apart from the discovery of novel mechanisms of action for Biz compounds, new initiatives must also be testified, such as personalized cancer chemotherapy (Lu et al., 2014), new pharmaceutical innovations (Ali 2011, Ali et al., 2011c) or drug combinations (Lu et al., 2014, Rhomberg et al., 2007). All these efforts will be not done in vain.

CONCLUSION

In this chapter, we address and highlight the different inhibitiory pathways against metastases *in vivo* and molecular mechanisms of action *in vitro* by Biz compounds, especially relating to the inhibitions of tumor metastasis including pathways of angiogenesis, topoisomerase II, calmodulin, sialic acid, fibrinogen, calmodulin, lipoperoxidation, GTPases, cell-movements and so on. We sincerely invite more money and attentions for deeper understanding of Biz compounds and create more useful clinical therapeutic strategies and drug combinations.

REFERENCES

Ali, I., et al. (2011a). Social aspects of cancer genesis. *Cancer Therapy*, *8*, 6-14.

Ali, I., et al. (2011b). Cancer scenario in India with future perspectives. *Cancer Therapy*, *8*, 56-70.

Ali, I., et al. (2011c). Advances in nano drugs for cancer chemotherapy, *Current Cancer Drug Targets*, *11*, 135-146.

Ali, I.. (2011). Nano anti-cancer drugs: Pros and cons and future perspectives, *Current Cancer Drug Targets*, *11*, 131-134.

Bakowski, M. T. (1976). ICRF 159. (+/-). 1, 2-di (3, 5-dioxopiperazin-1-yl). propane NSC-129, 943; razoxane. *Cancer Treat Rev.*, *3*, 95-107.

Barry, E., et al. (2008). Absence of secondary malignant neoplasms in children with high-risk acute lymphoblastic leukemia treated with dexrazoxane. *J Clinical Oncology.*, *26*, 1106-1111.

Bellet, R. E., et al. (1976). Phase II study of ICRF-159 in patients with metastatic colorectal carcinoma previously exposed to systemic chemotherapy. *Cancer Treat Rep.*, *60*, 1395-1397.

Bobek, V. (2012). Anticoagulant and fibrinolytic drugs—possible agents in treatment of lung cancer? *Anticancer Agents in Medicinal Chemistry*, *12*, 580-588.

Braybrooke, J. P. (2000). A phase II study of razoxane, an antiangiogenic topoisomerase II inhibitor, in renal cell cancer with assessment of potential surrogate markers of angiogenesis. *Clin. Cancer Res.*, *6*, 4697-4704.

Costantini, V., & Zacharski, L. R. (1992). The role of fibrin in tumor metastasis. *Cancer Metastasis Rev. 11*, 283-290.

Creighton, A. M., et al. (1969). Antitumour activity in a series of bisdiketopiperazines. *Nature*, *222*, 384-385.

Dvorak, H. F., et al. (1983). Fibrin as a component of the tumor stroma: origins and biological significance., *Cancer Metastasis Rev.*, *2* , 41-73.

Grint, T., et al. (2012). Fibrinogen—a possible extracellular target for inosital phosphates. *Messenger*, *1*, 160-166.

He, H., et al. (1988). Cytokinetic effects of 1, 2-bis (4-isobutoxycarbonyloxy-methyl-3, 5-dioxopiperazin-1-yl). ethane (MST-16). on leukemia L1210 cells in mice. *Acta Pharmacol Sin*, *9*, 369-373.

Hellmann, K. & Burrage, K. (1969). Control of malignant metastases by ICRF-159. *Nature.*, *224*, 273-275.

Hellmann, K. & Rhomberg, W. (1991). Radiotherapeutic enhancement by razoxane. *Cancer Treat Rev.*, *18*, 225-240.

Hellmann, K. (2003). Dynamics of tumor angiogenesis: effect of razoxane- induced growth rate slowdown. *Clin. Exp. Metastasis.*, *20*, 95-102.

Herman, E. H., et al. (1982)., Properties of ICRF-159 and related Bis(dioxopiperazine). compounds. *Advances in Pharmacology and Chemotherapy.*, Garattini S, Goldin A, Hawking F, Kopin IJ; Ed. New York; Academy Press 1982, Vol *19*, 249-290.

James, S. E. & Salsbury, A. J. (1974). Effect of (±).-1,2-bis(3,5-dioxopiperazin-1-yl). propane non tumor blood vessels and its relationship to the antimetastatic effect in the Lewis lung carcinoma. *Cancer Res.*, *34(4).*, 839-842.

Ji, RY. (1988). Probimane. *Drugs. Fut.*, *13*, 418-419.

Jones, J. M., et al. (2006). Plasma fibrinogen and serum C-reactive protein are associated with non-small cell lung cancer. *Lung Cancer*, *53*, 97-101.

Kane, R. C., et al. (2008). Dexrazoxane (Totect[TM]). FDA review and approval for the treatment of accidental extravasation following intravenous anthracycline chemotherapy. *The Oncologist.*, *13*, 445-450.

Lu, D. Y. & Cao, J. Y. (2001b). Structural aberration of cellular sialic acids and their functions in cancer., *J Shanghai Univ (Eng).*, *5*, 164-170.

Lu, D. Y. & Lu, T. R. (2010a). Anticancer activities and mechanisms of bisdioxopiperazine compounds probimane and MST-16. *Anti-cancer Agent Medicinal Chemistry.* *10*, 78-91.

Lu, D. Y. & Lu, T. R. (2010b). Antimetastatic activities and mechanisms of bisdioxopiperazine compounds. *Anti-Cancer Agent Medicinal Chemistry.* *10*, 564-570.

Lu, D. Y., et al. (1993). Distribution of ^{14}C labeled at dioxopiperazine or methyl morphorline group of probimane by whole body autoradiography. *Acta. Pharmacol. Sin.*, *14*, 171-173.

Lu, D. Y., et al. (1994). Serum contents of sialic acids in mice bearing different tumors. *Chin. Sci. Bull. (Eng).*, *39*, 1220-1223.

Lu, D. Y., et al. (1999). Comparison of some antineoplastic drugs on inhibiting thrombin catalyzing fibrinogen clotting in vitro. *Chin Med J (Eng).*, *112*, 1052-1053.

Lu, D. Y., et al. (2000). Effects of cancer chemotherapy on the blood fibrinogen concentrations of cancer patients. *J Int Med Res.*, *28*, 313-317.

Lu, D. Y., et al. (2001). Comparison between probimane and razoxane on inhibiting calmodulin activity of rabbit erythrocyte membrane. *Chin J Pharmacol Toxicol*, *15*, 76-78.

Lu, D. Y., et al. (2003)., The inhibition of probimane on lipoxidation of rabbit and human erythrocytes. *J Shanghai University (Engl).*, *7*, 301-304.

Lu, D. Y. et al. (2004a). Effect of anticancer drugs on the binding of ^{125}I-fibrinogen to two leukemia cell lines *in vitro*. *J. Int. Med. Res*, *32*, 488-491.

Lu, D. Y et al. (2004b). Anti-tumor effects of two bisdioxopiperazines against two experimental lung cancer models in vivo. *BMC Pharmacology. 4*, 32.

Lu, D. Y., et al. (2005). Anti-proliferative effects, cell cycle G_2/M phase arrest and blocking of chromosome segregation by probimane and MST-16 in human tumor cell lines., *BMC Pharmacology.*, *5*, 11.

Lu, D. Y., et al. (2006). Medicinal chemistry of probimane and MST-16: comparison of anticancer effects between bisdioxopiperazines. *Medicinal Chemistry. 2*, 369-375.

Lu, D. Y., et al. (2007a). Treatment of solid tumors and metastases by fibrinogen-targeted anticancer drug therapy. *Med Hypotheses.*, *68*, 188-193.

Lu, D. Y., et al. (2007b). Relationship between blood fibrinogen concentration and pathological features of cancer patients: a 139-case clinical study. *Online J Biological Science, 7*, 8-11.

Lu, D. Y., et al. (2007c). The antiproliferative effects of probimane and razoxane on tumor cells are concomitant with inhibition of hemolysis and calmodulin (CaM). action and a new CaM-ATPase acting model. *Res J Biol Sci.*, *2*, 127-133.

Lu, D. Y., et al. (2010a). Different spontaneous pulmonary metastasis inhibitions against Lewis lung carcinoma in mice by Bisdioxopiperazine compounds of different treatment schedules. *Sci Pharm, 78(1).* 13-20.

Lu, D. Y., et al. (2010b). The absorption, distribution and excretion of ^{14}C-probimane in mice bearing Lewis lung carcinoma. *Sci Pharm, 78*, 445-450.

Lu, D. Y., et al. (2010c). Cell manifestation of bisdioxopiperazines treatment of human tumor cells lines in culture. *Anti-Cancer Agent Medicinal Chemistry.*, *10*, 657-660.

Lu, D. Y., et al. (2011). Antimetastatic therapy targeting aberrant sialylation profiles in cancer cells. *Drug Therapy Studies, 1*, e12.

Lu, D. Y., et al. (2012). Development of antimetastatic drugs by targeting tumor sialic acids. *Sci Pharm, 80*, 497-508.

Lu, D. Y., et al. (2013a). Cancer metastases treatments. *Current Drug Therapy, 8*, 24-29.

Lu, D. Y., et al. (2013b). Inhibitions of some antineoplastic drugs on serum sialic acid levels in mice bearing tumors. *Sci Pharm, 81*, 223-231.

Lu, D. Y.,. (2014). Personalized cancer chemotherapy, an effective way for enhancing outcomes in clinics. Woodhead Publishing, Elsevier, UK.

Lu, D. Y., et al. (2015). Tumor fibrin/fibrinogen matrix as a unique therapeutic target for pulmonary cancer growth and metastases. *Clin Res Pulmonology.*, *3*, 1027.

O'connell, M. J. (1980). Randomized clinical trial comparing two dose regimens of ICRF-159 in refractory malignant lymphomas. *Cancer Treat Rep.*, *64*, 1355-1358.

Okamoto, T. et al. Long-term administration of oral low-dose topoisomerase II inhibitors, MST-16 and VP- 16, for refractory or relapsed non-Hodgkin's lymphoma. *Acta. Haematol., 2000*, *104*(2-3)., 128-130.

Polterauer, S., et al. (2009). Fibrinogen plasma levels are an independent prognostic parameter in patients with cervical cancer. *Am J Obstet Gynecol.*, *200*, 647.

Rhomberg, W., et al. (2007). Razoxane and vindesine in advanced soft tissue sarcomas: impact on metastasis survival and radiation response. *Anticancer Res, 27*, 3609-3614.

Salsbury, A. J., et al. (1974). Histological analysis of the antimetastatic effect of (±)-1,2-bis(3,5-dioxopiperazin-1-yl). propane. *Cancer Res, 34*, 843-849.

Siegel, R. L., et al. (2015). Cancer stastistics. *CA-Cancer J Clin. 65*, 5-29.

Valastyan S. & Weinberg R. A. (2011). Tumor metastasis: molecular insights and evolving paradigms. *Cell*, *147*, 275-292.

van Hille, B., et al. (2000). Characterization of the biological and biochemical activities of F 11782 and bisdioxopiperazine, ICRF-187 and ICRF-193, two types of topoisomerase II catalytic inhibitors with distinctive mechanisms of action. *Anti-cancer Drugs*, *11*, 829-841.

Varmus, H. (2006). The new era in cancer research. *Science*, *312*, 1162-1165.

Verheul, H. M. W. & Pinedo, H. M. (2007). Possible molecular mechanisms involved in the toxicity of angiogenesis inhibition. *Nature Rev Cancer*, *7*, 475-485.

Vuong, M. C., et al. (2013). A comparative study of the cytotoxic and genotoxic effects of ICRF-154 and bimolane, two catalytic inhibitors of topoisomerase II. *Mutations Res/Genetic Toxicology and Environmental mutagenesis.*, *750*, 63-71.

Wang, M. Y., et al.. (1988). Effects of bimolane and probimane on the incorporation of [3H]TdR, [3H]UR and [3H]Leu into Ehrlich ascites carcinoma cells in vitro. *Acta Pharmacol Sin*, *9*, 367-369.

Yang, K. Z., et al. (1990). Short-term results of malignant lymphoma treated with probimane. *Chin J Cancer*, *9*, 192-193.

INDEX

B

C

T

U